Genesis 22:17: I will indeed bless you and make your offspring as numerous as the stars of the sky and the sand on the seashore. Your offspring will possess the gates of their enemies. (HCS)

Hardcover ISBN 978-1-957077-73-4
Softcover ISBN 978-1-957077-74-1

Cover image: Shutterstock JAG-cz

HARVEST OF HEALING, LLC

Izauh 61™

Publishing assistance by BookCrafters, Parker, Colorado.
www.bookcrafters.net

In an Attempt to Save the World

HOME-MADE ANSWERS FOR CANCER
And Life Altering Disease

A Personal Journey With a Positive Outcome

HARVEST OF HEALING, LLC

Izauh 61™

PREFACE

Life experiences produce wisdom; textbooks produce knowledge.

To comprehend the work product presented herein, a person must realize that at times there is no logical explanation for how or why events occur, you just have to ride with the facts that unfold. Here is where the terms Mother Nature, God or Universe fit in. An increasing amount of events that unfold in life simply have no logical explanation. One must learn to accept the unexplainable in an attempt to unravel a seemingly unchangeable situation. This is where I should insert my phrase: Trusting and Believing Have Been Contaminated by a Desire to Understand. It is somewhat of a challenge to attempt to project a big picture when there are many factors at play. The attempt is to bring the factors of these unexplainable events to a connection point where they develop into an understandable outcome.

This book is set out in two parts. Part 1 describes my personal health journey that took on many twists and turns throughout my life. Much of my journey was spent like many others, trying to find answers in the common places. A few breakthroughs were experienced yet my health would cycle back into the unexplainable reactions that would not go away. I have never been overweight. Smoking and alcoholic beverages were never an interest for me. I practiced good eating habits, proper hygiene and my house was always clean, quite clean in fact. None of the common risk factors overshadowed me like smoking, drinking or eating unhealthy.

I share my personal journey through health challenges to enlighten the reader and hopefully researchers, with respect to gaps in modern day testing and treatment. I raise a flag in an attempt to bring rescue from the downward spiral called "disease" crouching over all. My hope is my story and the wisdom I have gained throughout my journey will resonate with others and bring inspiration. Once I realized the "how and why" of where most of my health issues originated, I began to dig deeper to find the potential initial triggers. I have always had this resounding belief that people were not created to be sickly or unhealthy. There is some root cause for the progressive downward motion in health that is prevalent today. If you fail to remove the root of the weed, the weed will keep sprouting back up.

If you are a person who processes concepts or ideas strictly on logic alone, this book is not for you. There are no laboratory test results, nor scientific discoveries, other than my own personal blood analysis, and genetic panel. Science has not contributed to my conclusions, nor did any other professional industry. Thus, any hard proof you may want does not exist other than my own personal health improvement, which only those close to me have witnessed. In part, my journey brought an entirely new perspective on life and opened my eyes to errors and gaps in formulas used by laboratories and industries to draw their professional conclusions. These incorrect or missing pieces can lead to destructive consequences when it comes to health.

As you will see in Part 1, my life contained many challenges that at times seemed unreal. A part of me wishes they had been unreal yet a part of me knows that I would not have the level of wisdom I own today had it not been for the various challenges, experiences, opportunities for researching numerous topics, and encounters with many people I crossed paths with along the way. For this I am grateful.

Part 2 of this book attempts to describe and potentially expose initiating points for disease. Origination of destruction, whether in health or in the condition of the earth, have come from historical events and modern day traditions that often result in the birth of a particular atmosphere and thus influencing the interior complex workings of the physical body. Descriptions are provided that unfold the possible inlets for the decline not only witnessed within the borders of the United States but around the world. I apply a broad perspective to attempt to capture the fine connecting threads that weave together each event or inlet. My hope is to assist in the ability to develop a new perspective that will bring forth the health humanity and the earth desperately need. The resulting atmosphere from traditions and customs can influence the physical body and when exposure to damaging atmospheres repeatedly take place it can result in unrecognizable changes within the body.

Cancer

Cancer is a collective disease. There is no individual food or toxin that is 100% guilty of causing cancer. Each individual person has a different risk level dependent upon the lifestyle of their ancestors and the individual exposure they themselves have encountered. In my personal situation, the door for cancer was opened through ancestors whose diet included consumption of yeast breads and honey that eventually produced bacteria in the blood that is unidentified even today. Elimination of the Ancient practices that protect the body from infection was also a contributor.

There are many contributing co-factors to cancer. Ancestors who worked in toxic environments, to those who had a medical condition that required an excessive amount of prescription medication, to those who were alcoholics, all of which has some level of a contributing factor. Couple any of these foundational, underlying factors with the level of toxins, chemicals, herbicides, pesticides, EMF/EMR, static electricity, and so on, people are exposed to today and it is no surprise cancer and other debilitating health issues are on the rise.

INDEX OF CONTENTS

PART 1

JOURNEY OF A LIFE TIME

Deuteronomy 5:33: Follow the whole instruction the Lord your God has commanded you, so that you may live, prosper, and have a long life in the land you possess. (HCS)

Many will agree that there are far too many incidents of life being cut short due to various reasons, foremost being from cancer or other life threatening disease. At the time of this writing, many people in the age range of 60 to 70 have lost their lives in the past 12-24 months. It is evident the age range for death due to disease is declining. The human race is on a slippery slope gliding ever so quickly to the cemetery plot! The continuing question is why? With the advancements in research, medical care and scientific discoveries, why are so many people, particularly those at an age of less than 50, encountering life threatening health challenges? What has gone wrong? What is to blame?

Life bounced me into the "learn as you go" program due to numerous voids for answers to the health concerns that plagued me. I learned I would need to read my body from the inside out on my own and couple it with a lot of faith! At times it seemed I was continually hitting roadblocks and a sense of no hope for gain would surround me. Nevertheless, I pushed forward, some days with eager anticipation and some days with none.

1 John 2:27: The anointing you received from Him remains in you, and you don't need anyone to teach you. Instead, His anointing teaches you about all things and is true and is not a lie; just as He has taught you, remain in Him. (HCS)

I would ask the "what is wrong" and "what is to blame" questions as I battled my way through numerous health disturbances throughout all of my childhood and most, well perhaps all, of my adult life until recently. Born with an inability to tolerate milk my upset tummy would no doubt cause me to excessively cry. Breast milk was my diet but my Mom would consume milk herself from the dairy cows my parents owned and the residual influence of the milk would come through to me. Eventually the pediatrician suggested I be given Pet Milk.

Elementary School lunches were a new found problem growing up at a time when "drink all your milk" was the golden rule. This golden rule resulted in a weekly upset tummy for me. Abdominal pains would last for a few hours. Additionally, as a child I had what was categorized as typical health setbacks such as swollen tonsils, sore throat, earaches, postnasal drip and continuing digestive upsets. The practice was to seek advice and treatment from Western Medicine practicing physicians during these flare-ups and work through any remaining symptoms the best you could. Many trips were made to the local physician's office sitting in the waiting room hunched over Mom's lap while waiting for my name to be paged. Back through the long hallway I'd go to hear the doctor once again instruct me to "say ahhhh" and report that my throat and ears were red. The ordered remedy was a penicillin shot, with a lollipop as the reward once the shot was concluded. Time and time again all the way through High School and early adult years this process was repeated. No explanation as to why the "infection" would repeat, it was just the way it was, or a "bug" you likely picked up at school.

Dental visits were all too common, none of which I cared for. Stomach pain would ensue and crying while in the dental chair was an every visit occurrence. I was traumatized by the process used to numb, drill and fill my teeth with mercury fillings in order "to avoid getting cavities," which was the common practice. The terror of dental offices plagued me into my adulthood. These experiences go into a category of "should have never taken place!"

As an adult, the swollen tonsils and sore throats continued and, by my early 20s, I traveled to a well-known allergy clinic for testing. The list of pollen allergies was quite long and the prescribed remedy was injections to assist in the symptoms experienced. Living in a rural community, it is impossible to avoid the weeds and dust so, at this stage, I was happy to have some form of relief from allergy symptoms.

Life in general was pretty plain and simple for me. I worked outside of the home for several years and eventually life required moving to another state where the climate was a little different. I was able to stop the use of the allergy injections and my health seemed pretty well balanced for a time.

The Summer of 1996, at the age of 33 I became quite ill which prompted a trip to the physician's office. I knew this episode of sore throat was much different than those of the past and fatigue was horrible! I inquired of the physician whether I could be experiencing Mononucleosis. The physician seemed to think my question was quite humorous telling me I would have had Mono when I was "much" younger and sent me on my way with a 5-day Z-Pack antibiotic. By day 2-3 of the medication my symptoms were continuing to worsen so back to the physician's office I went. This time blood was collected for various types of testing, some of which the doctor suggested should be for cancer. Great! I returned home to wait 10 days for blood analysis conclusions and the physician's office to call. That was a long 10 days even when I was sleeping through most of it. I arrived at my appointment for the doctor to review the test results and much to his surprise, I had an active case of Mononucleosis/Epstein Barr Virus (EBV) at, in his words, "levels he had never seen before." His suggested treatment was for me to go home and go to bed.

At this point there wasn't much else I could do. The glands in my neck were so swollen I could not turn my head causing people to think I had been in a car accident or something. My skin was yellow from the stress on my liver, and to be honest, a daily shower took more energy than what I had, often putting me right back in the bed I had just removed myself from. Late June through late August was spent at home in bed. By late Summer I had returned to work, although it was a challenge due to lingering fatigue and headaches. Insomnia now dominated my nights. Every natural remedy to ease the sleepless nights was of no success and often resulted in some form of allergic reaction. Everything from essential oil, to warm baths, to soothing candle scents and relaxing environments, you name it, I tried it and none of it worked. Years later I would wonder if a genetic mutation from EBV could result in descendants having insomnia. Herein may be an answer to the insomnia many battle today.

Years progressed with new symptoms and more trips to the physician's office. I figured out by this point that when a physician didn't seem to have an explanation for the symptoms on display they would tell me I had a virus. There were times I was offered prescription pain medications but I refused them all. My body did not tolerate prescriptions of any type very well and particularly not pain medications. It was not my desire to have issues covered up, I wanted them identified and eliminated. By this point I decided the "figuring it out and the process of knowing how to eliminate it" became my job.

In 2004 after an extended trip overseas I arrived back into the United States with what I thought was horrible jet lag. After attempting to recover with just rest for about a week and there being no relief, back to the physician's office I went. Blood analysis was done and the conclusion was Chronic Fatigue and Fibromyalgia. A prescription was offered but declined since the prescribed drug had a side effect of Schizophrenia. I decided I did not need to add that possibility to the mix of health issues I was already experiencing. I wanted a cure, not a bandage for the issues. This system of diagnosing and having no form of option or plan to eliminate the "diagnosis" was becoming frustrating for me. I refused to settle for being labeled with anything. My goal was "identify" the disruption and repair it, not cover it up.

My time was now spent on researching topics related to Chronic Fatigue; a monthly massage appointment, weekly chiropractic adjustments, and frequent acupuncture sessions. What could be going on inside of me and who was out there to help me? I came across a book titled From Fatigue to Fantastic, which then led me to a local physician who conducted tests and concluded that I was suffering from Heavy Metal Toxicity.

Part of 2005 was spent undergoing weekly IV therapy to assist in the removal of various heavy metals that had accumulated in my body. The IV therapy resulted in an entirely new set of reactive symptoms. My muscles would feel as though they were set in concrete, rock hard yet squeezing me and painful. I can only relate this to a feeling one might get when falling and the reaction is to tense up. This would last for a few hours and often the only relief I found was by sitting in hot bathwater to attempt to relieve the pain. The treating physician gave no concern for my reaction to the therapy and discounted the episodes as merely "detoxing." Again, my question was, how does a person get Heavy Metal Toxicity and why is my body responding in a negative way to the therapy? I didn't work or live in any heavily toxic environment. This is when I began to learn about the dangers of car exhaust, aluminum baking pans and beverage containers, and mercury fillings. These revelations led to an entirely new set of obstacles. Aluminum pans were replaced and I ate nothing that even came near aluminum foil remembering the days when my Mom would cook the Sunday roast wrapped in foil. I drank nothing from an aluminum can and headed to the dentist to get mercury fillings replaced that had been initiated during my childhood and early adult years. After removal of the common culprits you would think my body would feel great. Nope. I concluded the IV therapy for Heavy Metal Toxicity after 45 treatments, many hours and several dollars later, none of which was covered by health insurance. I still felt horrible. I concluded the therapy with a continual vapor of no energy and feeling flu-like, yet apparently free of excessive harmful metals.

Amongst my travel through IV therapy for Heavy Metal Toxicity I landed at the local Ear Nose and Throat (ENT) specialist's office with uncontrollable swollen tonsils. My tonsils had been problematic since I was a child. The ENT specialist confirmed my tonsils were infected. Several months later I would come to realize the infection was Candida related. It was advised the only remedy was to have my tonsils removed. Having the tonsils removed was one of the most painful experiences I had encountered and that is coming from someone who is no sissy when it comes to pain levels. My body does not tolerate Tylenol well simply due to the stress it puts on the liver yet I was informed that Tylenol was the only form of pain relief the specialist would prescribe for after surgery care. The need for some form of pain relief was great so I took the Tylenol for what little pain relief it seemed to provide. I experienced nights of being unable to sleep because of the stress on my liver. This was an eventful experience and one I'm glad I will never have to experience again. It did raise a question about the level of function of my lymph system. Tonsils are a part of the lymph system and why was my lymph unable to process and eliminate the waste it needed to?

Around this time I invested in an ion footbath unit, which I still use today. The unit assists the lymph by removing some of the toxic load the body is attempting to process. Again, like a toddler who constantly asks questions, I want to know what has caused the lymph system to become so sluggish. By this time you would think that I would have figured out that with each question God will grant an experience that results in the answer! Having gained a little insight on Symbolic representations, more on Symbols in Part 2, Language of the Cosmos, sitting in pools of water, like in a bathtub or even a lake, produces a signal to the cells of non-moving water, that which is still. The lymph must process toxic debris through movement of fluid. A genetic mutation for lymph related issues was birthed through sitting in a bath or other form of stationary water.

By this point in time medical professionals began to discount my symptoms and place me in a category of one who likes to be sick or wants attention. Medical testing indicated I did not have depression and their conclusion that I wanted to be sick was, and still is, far from who I am or what I wanted. I wanted to be well, to feel well and have an ability to function through a day without encountering a major setback. It was difficult to plan any event in advance simply because there was no way to calculate which day I would feel well enough to travel or be in public.

In the Fall of 2008, while watching the television show Mystery Diagnosis, I recognized a photo of a bulls-eye bite wound that had been identified as a tick bite on a young teenage girl who had experienced debilitating fatigue, joint aches, and so on. I felt for this young girl as I had experienced the same symptoms that were described in her story. By the end of this episode, I was convinced that yet another underlying health issue had to be from a tick bite from years prior. In the early 1990s I returned home from a camping trip with a bulls-eye shaped rash on my left shoulder. When the local physician was consulted I was given a topical ointment and told the bite was "not spider" related. The revelation received through the Mystery Diagnosis broadcast initiated my quest to locate a physician that would properly test for and treat Lyme's Disease with a therapy that had a holistic approach. I had success at finding a physician and began treatment for the three Lyme's bacteria, out of a possible four, that reflected in the blood test. Part of my treatment program included an oral antibiotic at 875 mg twice per day in addition to a prescription that worked at amplifying the effectiveness of the antibiotic. Vitamin supplements and hormone therapy were implemented to assist in balancing and general recovery. I coupled the treatment plan with a form of energy/meridian therapy, far infrared sauna, ion footbath therapy and massage. Within four months, a repeated blood test came back negative for Lyme's.

Although the Lyme's infection was no longer present, vapors from chemicals, including perfumes and scented candles gave me a headache and caused my sinuses to burn; condensed areas of power lines or power substations made my thyroid visibly quiver; a massage began to make me feel as though I had consumed a Grande coffee! This is just a tip to the iceberg of symptoms I would encounter. Medical professionals thought this is something I desired? There is only one logical explanation for why I was categorized in such a manner: they did not have appropriate knowledge to identify or treat what was taking place inside of me. There is still much room for improvement in the realms of medical treatment.

Once the therapies for Lyme's were complete I began a four month Candida Cleanse Diet to assist in eliminating Candida yeast build up as a result of being on antibiotics for an extended period of time. The physician promises continued, that I would feel much better after the yeast was cleared out of my body. Many promises for improvement were extended throughout my journey but I was having difficulty achieving the improvement promised! I lost count of how many times I was assured I would feel better after a particular regimented therapy. None of the physicians wanted to believe me when I would share with them that my body does not respond well to the printed and established guidelines followed by physicians. Numerous times my body resisted the standard treatment seemingly resulting in the medical standards being incorrect, incomplete or, one would hate to assume, a hoax.

After making my way through 20 years of Lyme's Disease, to the Summer of 1996 being spent in bed with Epstein Barr Virus and Mononucleosis at levels "never seen" before by the treating physician, I felt fried! Many years followed with attempts to manage the cascading health influences each of those infections, let alone having them at the same time, have on a physical body (Note: EBV can be inherited through DNA). I have been Lyme's Disease free for 16 years and counting, something medical professionals told me was not possible. After consulting medical professionals for the numerous health threats and challenges I was experiencing and receiving little aid from the then available printed and taught remedies, by 2015/2016 I was on a fast track to a cancer diagnosis.

During my journey, there were times I would be advised to take a multi-vitamin and sometimes it would be suggested that I increase a specific vitamin or mineral. My body promptly told me it did not like multi-vitamins. I chalked this up to my body being unable to handle receiving so much information at one time. When I took B Complex supplements, supposedly for energy, my body would become fatigued. A few family members are the same in this category. Calcium and/or Magnesium would cause my legs to feel restless, no matter what type of calcium or magnesium I took. So what is it in the chemical reactions category that is taking place in my blood that is so different than the majority of the population? By this point, my conclusion was the "one size fits all" approach does not always fit "all."

In the Fall of 2020 a new set of symptoms erupted that initiated the need for a genetic analysis. The genetic analysis revealed a condition of hyperactive inflammation response, which has been given a label of Mast Cell Activation Syndrome. I immediately began following a low-histamine diet regimen, coupled with a variety of supplements and custom herbs. Thanks to the Nutritionist consulted, the herbs and low-histamine diet brought some relief.

My senses persisted that there was a deeper issue. What was causing this inflammation issue and how did the genetic mutations come about? Again, the medical professionals consulted seemed oblivious to the mystery within me and made no note of the increasing white blood cell count reflected in my yearly blood analysis. I was simply informed that my blood work "looked great," even though my body felt as though it was dying. After a few months of debilitating health symptoms and frustration with the path I was attempting to walk along with healthcare, I decided it was time to investigate and make changes once again on my own.

By mid-2021 I had been on a low-histamine diet for approximately six months and continued to gather information that developed into additional changes in the way I did things in everyday life. My lifestyle, clothing choices, hygiene, diet, environment, priorities, sleeping habits, hobbies and activities all took on a different shape and meaning. After implementing the "all things new and different," a blood analysis in August 2022 reflected the white blood cell count that had steadily increased over the prior three years had decreased by one-half in just a matter of nine months. I was able to begin tapering off the herbal supplements.

Needless to express, my eyes were opened to some flaws and missing components in relation to laboratory conclusions and industries practices, and not just the medical industry. My life had to change in order to regain any form of good health. The lifestyle changes implemented are what I share in this book.

3 John 1:2: Dear friend, I pray that you may enjoy good health and that all may go well with you, even as your soul is getting along well. (NIV) (emphasis added)

PART 2

INTRODUCTION

The Human Race has been set upon a path that will lead to its extinction if the captain of the Human Race ship called Humanity is not replaced. Who is in charge? And who should be in charge? These are the questions to ask.

The level of incident of debilitating disease, crippling influence and even death of generations that should be thriving is on the rise. When conversations focus on 20 and 30 year old persons who lack an ability to function through a day as a consequence of a debilitating disease or illness, or have been led down a path of unchangeable influence called cancer, there are serious problems with the way life is being lived. The Human Race has come to the point it is planting weed seeds, (meaning contaminated DNA), rather than healthy, vibrant offspring.

Healthcare providers spend a great deal of time swatting at the flies that breed, swarm and infest the physical body, in part due to a lack of ability to keep up with what is actually taking place inside the body. Fifty years ago life didn't require the amount of time and money now spent by the average person on attempting to maintain their health.

In June 2024 a quick Google search revealed the following statistics for 2024:

66% of U.S. adults take prescription drugs;
65% of those in Canada take prescription drugs;
35% of those in Australia take prescription drugs; and
26% of U.K. adults take prescription drugs.

More than 39 million people around the world have drug use disorders. (SingleCare.com)

As a race, we were originally designed to thrive. At this point in time, many, quite possibly the majority of persons lack the ability to thrive. Living life with vitality no longer exists. The original design did not include the necessity of prescription drugs, or synthetic supplements that can often be a mockery of authentic nutrients, yet sold and labeled for consumption. Temporary bandages are applied to serious health issues for the person to be able to function through a day. This, I say, is not life as it was intended to be. People are moving in a direction that will produce future generations of even shorter life spans; the ability to live and function beyond 40 or even 50 years old will not exist. Moving in this direction for a few generations will eventually lead to extinction.

It is not only the typical culprits of smoking, consumption of alcohol or a fast food diet that has contributed to the problem. One way people can invite their own demise is simply by the materials and design they cover their body in everyday that has been grossly mislabeled as fashionable clothing. There are universal guidelines and restrictions for clothing if one desires to live healthy. The body cannot be clothed in chemically made materials and be expected to be disease or health disruption free. The fashion industry appears to be just as guilty as the food industry, the chemical and toxins industries, the medical industry, and so forth. More details on this subject will follow.

The light (electricity) within blood cells has diminished due to numerous contaminates encountered not only by those living today, but by their ancestors who set the cells of the body in motion for disease. The Human Race must take action to recapture optimum health.

Do those in positions of authority lack the level of wisdom it would take to set the current wheels that are progressing toward destruction back into their proper place? Money and power seem to be the focus of many of those positioned at the controls of those wheels, rather than rearing up generations that will aid in the care of older generations and simply having an ability to introduce healthy new generations. The Human Race has a noose around its neck, often labeled as some form of common practice, belief or custom, tradition, standard, or the insurance coverage any of those things do business with.

If Humans were thriving there would not be the great need for healthcare we see today in its numerous and various forms. Humans must step off of this Merry-Go-Round of destruction if they are to exist in the future with any form of functionality. Humankind has been bounced into a position of maintaining to get through a day rather than living with vitality that would benefit the Human Race and also planet earth herself. If you doubt this conclusion, read the Book of Genesis and the assignment given to Adam. Adam's original assignment did not involve a form of strenuous manual labor but an existence that brought life to him and his surroundings. How is this done? Through the atoms that make up the cells. Similar to a cell phone that has been misused, abused or hacked, so are the cells of the human body. The manual labor for Adam came after the words of the snake in the tree led him and his female companion, Eve, astray. Following the advice of the snake, a voice that should not be listened to, caused Adam to be removed from the life of a flourishing garden to a life of struggle. Where is the Symbol of a snake commonly seen today? In a nutshell, this is what has taken place and where Humankind is today.

There is only one Source that is capable of regulating, protecting and causing the condition of vitality and that Source governs the cosmos. When given the proper tools and equipment, that form of governing power will transform and protect the human body at the cellular level. The issue now becomes being aware of and educated in those specific tools and equipment.

When the Human Race is in the position of producing "Life with Vitality," planet earth will also thrive and the momentum behind "Save the Whales" or "Save a Tree/Rain Forest" will fade. The laws of natural order will thrive. In order to return to the position of thriving the Handbook for Life with Vitality must be properly followed. This Handbook, through the years, has been revised, stripped of its value, altered in many ways and even in some instances thrown out of the archives of "Important." The paths that have led to disease and destruction were put into place long ago by these alterations. If there was, or still is, any purposely planned destruction of the Human Race in place by those alive on this earth today, may God's hand be against them and their plans.

A cry is being sent forth for the Ancient Ways set forth in the Handbook for Life and the truth within its instruction to be put into place. This Handbook for Life is often called the Holy Bible. Before the publication of the Holy Bible (first published in approximately 1611), there was and still is today, the Bhagavad Gita of India, the sacred Scripture that was written thousands of years ago. In its entirety, the Holy Bible gives instructions on how to care for the body, how to live healthy and productive lives, how the forces that govern the cosmos can aid, or even harm the physical body.

The gossip that has been produced from the misinterpretation of the Handbook is a contributor to the path of destruction the generations are currently on. The Truth must be told, honored and practiced in order for the Humanity ship we are traveling on to be turned around!

Chapter I

LIVING IN UNISON WITH THE ENERGY

Jeremiah 6:16: This is what the Lord says: Stand by the roadways and look. Ask about the Ancient paths: which is the way to what is good? Then take it and find rest for yourselves. But they protested. "We won't." (HCS)

Energy can be described in many different ways. The dictionary definition of Energy: vigorous action; effort; the capacity for action or performance; usable power (as heat or electricity); the resource for producing such power. Words that relate to Energy: Force, main, might, muscle, potency, power, strength, vigor, life, pep, and vitality.

In the following chapters I make reference to Star Dust, a term I shared in the book From Antichrist to I AM published by Harvest of Healing, LLC in the Spring of 2022. Star Dust is a term I chose to represent the light or electrical activity that comes from the cosmos to the blood cells. Star Dust, through years of exposure to various elements, has become lost or depleted.

I also reference Energy, being a form of electrical charge produced in and by the cosmic atmosphere and received through the cells in our body, when circumstances allow.

Through the passage of time a shift in the atmosphere has occurred. This shift is quite obvious and the results are evident in the activities of nature that produce torrential rains, storms of fire, unusual winds, increase in strength of hurricanes and tornadoes. This shift has also contributed to a hindered ability for the blood cells within our body to receive adequate signals from the cosmos in order to maintain their proper function. The Mayans may have been correct, the "end of the world" as we know it, seems to have arrived. These events are beyond the sphere of global warming. Things currently being classified as a result of global warming would not be taking place if there were not some form of electrical or magnetic event fueling them. The earth herself is stressed!

Humanity has also witnessed the shift through an increase in viral infections, fungal and bacterial occurrences. It makes the mind wonder how and why did this shift, that appears to be leading to an ultimate destruction, begin to take place? Yes, pollution is a big contributor, but let's look beyond the pollution. It appears we (humanity and the earth herself) are headed for a crash landing, an extinction of sorts. How does humanity go about turning the tide of Energy around in a beneficial, prosperous direction?

I confess to NOT being a Scientist, Biologist, Chemist or any other form of educated guru. What I will admit is my experiences and revelations point to some contributory factors that are leading mankind and the earth to complete destruction. Possibly, in years to come, someone wearing a white lab jacket will obtain an explanation for what I share that may be a bit more tangible for the human mind. For now, I will work with what I have, setting forth a pathway that future minds, geniuses or entrepreneurs can piece together.

Basics

While it is easy for me to unload information on how things called life began in a downward spiral, my typical "keep it simple" approach is not always understood by those not accustomed to this style. I ask for pardon if details are lacking. It is likely those details have been chalked up to the "everyone already knows this" category. Too much detail can become cumbersome, too little leaves one in doubt and disbelief. In part, the ability to grasp what is being said will depend on what era one comes from. The up and coming generations will grasp the concepts much easier than those who were born prior to say the 1960s. It has nothing to do with intelligence, it has to do with how life has been lived and what has been taught and accepted as truth.

Many components I share can be connected back to illustrations present throughout Ancient Text, hymns or myths, and Scripture contained in the Holy Bible, all of which are connected by threads, some are just simply written in contrasting types and styles of communication. Symbolic representations are common in Ancient Text and can be a challenge to interpret. (More on Symbols in Chapter IV, Language of the Cosmos.)

Stories get passed down through generations and a word or name becomes changed, a meaning of a word may shift for cultural reasons and after a period of time, the story becomes altered. It becomes like the old children's game Telephone. The first person receives a word then passes it to the next; the second person repeats the word to the third person, and so forth along the line until the last person announces the word they heard, often times resulting in the initial word having no relation to the final word shared.

History

Scanning through "once upon a time," life in general that was lived 400, 500 and even 1,000 years ago displayed an entirely different picture than what is seen today. Families generally lived secluded lives, grew their own food, and had little interaction with anyone outside of their family. Attire was of a specific style and made of natural fabrics, all of natural colors. There were no chemicals applied to crops; food was fresh, nothing prepackaged or made by someone else (exclusive of a few rare occasions), meals were kept fairly simple, and cool water was used to rid bacteria. Bathtubs made their debut in the 1800s. Prior to that time bathing was not an act of sitting in a stationary pool of warm water. Listening to music was rare and only created through certain instruments, and certainly not pumped through amplifiers or speakers. Life was fairly simplistic. Yes, it was hard work bucketing water, growing food and preparing meals on an open fire or wood-burning stove. The presence of a harmful environment was quite limited.

I am not suggesting modern day conveniences must be removed to bring humanity and the earth back into alignment with the proper Energy. What I am attempting to relay is that when the lifestyle of the Ancient past in general is viewed and compared to the lifestyle of the current day SOMETHING, many things, initiated a shift in the level and quality of Energy that should exist in human lives.

Why Are We On Earth?

Let's look at "In The Beginning" once again. This may be a leap for some but hang in there with me as I drive to a point.

Genesis 1 is the story of the steps taken by God (the main Energy source) to create and supply the earth. Day, night, plants, animals, all come on the scene. Then with everything set in place on the earth, God creates man (meaning the physical body), IN HIS IMAGE references the human body has a capacity to generate or contain a copy of the Energy that is sometimes called "God" or "Creator." What was the physical body to do with this Energy?

Genesis 1:26: ...and let them (mankind) have dominion over the fish of the sea, and over the fowl of the air and over the cattle, and over all the earth, and over every creeping thing that creepeth upon the earth. (NIV) (emphasis and notation added)

In a nutshell, the Energy carried by humans will determine the health and wellbeing of themselves and of the earth and everything within it. Many activities, or lack thereof, of mankind, has resulted in the decline of life and vitality. Much has suffered including vegetation, air quality and weather patterns. Instead of a flourishing life, we have now birthed viruses, beetle infestations, pollution and the list continues. The current approach to saving whales and rain forests will not correct the issues at hand. While those things play their part they are not a source of correction that will bring ultimate change to the earth as a whole.

Mankind must learn how to live in a way that produces a positive, life-giving Energy so the earth will respond in a way that becomes evident. Vegetation will flourish, animals will display a less aggressive or less timid demeanor; unruly viruses, fungus, bacteria and parasites will diminish.

The filament, I will call it, inside a cell must be properly charged with the Star Dust. When that filament receives the proper electrical charge, similar to a light bulb, the body will be healthy and share its "light" with the environment and ultimately the earth.

Humanity has evolved into a pattern of life and daily activities that produce dominatingly harmful environments. Such an environment has reached a level where viruses, whether new strains or reoccurrence of prior strains, and other infectious components have increased greatly over the past 100 or so years. We are a species that has and continues to create or allow, our own demise. The answers for how to correct the direction in which life is going are held within Ancient Text, and not in a laboratory or classroom. Let's ponder that for a moment.

Did humans create the COVID virus? Yes, but not just one human, all humans collectively. How? Because humans have not had the proper degree of electrical charge to do their earth cleaning job sufficiently. At the end of the day, it does not matter where the virus first became evident or who got their hands on it first. The bigger issue is WHY was COVID (or any plague) birthed; what caused it to come into being, along with all of the other infectious organisms. My thought: The chemical components within the body are no longer in the proper proportions necessary to maintain the electrical element(s) needed. The blood cells have lost the appropriate level of electrical charge allowing for opportunistic organisms to arise. Not only can the optimum charge help keep the physical body free from disease but it can also slow or stop the production of infectious components. Elevated occurrence of specific vibrations can brew up an atmosphere for infectious components.

The damage done has not been and will not be corrected by any group or individual meditation, yoga class, spiritual gathering, religion, or by singing Kumbaya. The falling away from health and vitality for all continues downward, evidence that these supposed remedies (yoga, religion, meditation, etc.) are not much, if any, help in correcting the bigger issue. In fact, participation in some of these activities can increase the momentum toward demise.

When an action is taken (exercise, meditation, and so on) there is a reaction that occurs. An Ancient Scripture states: <u>People perish for their lack of knowledge</u>. Truly, the knowledge that maintains life has been lost.

Not every human will be onboard with what it will require to cause change. But, when enough people who hold the correct genetics/DNA within their blood join forces in living life according to Ancient instruction, the vitality of humanity and the earth will turn around.

God-Creator is the power station; people with the correct blood components can become sub-stations!

What Creates Life-Giving Energy?

There is a lifestyle that resurrects an Ancient genetic code that has been lost through the sands of time. Hundreds of years ago there was a specific group of people that held the keys to influencing the environment around them, and within them and others. This genetic code has been depleted, though in some cases not completely erased, through events of history, foods, synthetic fibers, chemicals, medical intervention and lifestyle choices. A part of this lifestyle includes the ability to connect with the cosmos in order to receive the required electrical charge that takes up residence within the cells. When the appropriate collections of people take the necessary steps the genetic code will be resurrected in its full capacity and evidence of a shift in the earth and amongst people will become apparent. Long ago these people who held the genetic keys were called Wise Women and Wise Men. Not everyone qualifies for such position. The qualification lies within the codes captured in the blood. The protocols I share will aid in the creation of the life-giving Energy.

Chapter II

WE MUST DECIDE IT'S OKAY TO NOT BE "NORMAL"

An individual who experiences loss of energy, restlessness, a feeling of being uneasy or uncomfortable in certain surroundings, insomnia or many other symptoms often gets put into a category of "not normal." What if their symptoms are a normal reaction?

When you place a person who has an elevated level of Star Dust into a material world, that person will have reactions or symptoms to the environment he/she is exposed to, simply because of the internal conflict between the worldly elements and the Star Dust. The filament inside the blood cells becomes endangered. Attempts to cause the person to be "more normal," or have less response to the clash of elements taking place, risks depleting the level of Star Dust. Essentially, attempts to change a symptom or eliminate the occurring reactions could very likely remove all spirit sensitivity and eventually produce a solely material body.

A body with an elevated level of Star Dust will not function in the material world in a like manner as a body with a low or no level of Star Dust. They cannot and frankly should not. A cosmic created electrical charge does not adapt to a material environment. When you attempt this, the Star Dust level depletes and when pushed too far can die off. Flipping this around, the same goes for physical/material bodies. A physical body cannot and will not be present in the cosmic atmosphere or "Heavens"; it does not and could not survive. Astronauts are a good example of how much effort it takes for a human to leave earth. There is much training, preparation and protective gear put in place before humans can launch off for the moon!

A person must begin to identify what is causing a reaction and why a physical reaction is occurring. Many times my body would give off a signal of nervousness or a feeling of being anxious. A good example of this is while riding in a vehicle if my travel took me past an electrical substation my thyroid would visibly quiver. I knew I was exposed to an opposing influence but attempting to figure out if I needed medical attention or if simply removing myself from the harmful environment would solve the problem was often a challenge. Over time I learned how to remove myself from the afflicting environment or issue and allow my body to process what it had come in contact with. Many nights were spent with the inability to fall asleep or stay asleep simply because of the adjustment the cells in my body had to make to erase the opposition encountered. Apostle Paul speaks of his encounters with dangerous or threatening situations in 2 Corinthians.

2 Corinthians 11:26-27: On frequent journeys, I faced dangers from rivers, dangers from robbers, dangers from my own people, dangers from the Gentiles, dangers in the city, dangers in the open country, dangers on the sea, and dangers among false brothers; labor and hardship, many sleepless nights, hunger and thirst, often without food, cold, and lacking clothing. (HCS)

God gave us symptoms or signals for a reason. Something as simple as the color of your clothing, the cell phone you carry or pick up multiple times per day, or the combination of food you eat during a day can all result in a symptom. Bright lights, sunlight and just plain noise can all trigger a symptom. Once a person learns to identify a reaction vs. a need for medical intervention, the less trips they will need to make to the physician's office. This skill takes time to learn.

Instead of attempting to change the way a person displays a reaction, a more beneficial plan of action may be to learn to observe the surroundings and allow the body to calm the symptom by adjusting the environment, food or clothing in their daily lives.

I can reassure you there is absolutely nothing "wrong" with over-reactive or overly sensitive people when the reaction is a result of an electrical processing hiccup in the body. The person must learn how to safely live in a material world, to reduce symptoms and protect the Star Dust. Some people are like a sponge and soak up all the opposing electrical activity around them, then have to figure out how to wring it all out!

We should not be motivated to deplete Star Dust but share with others how they might increase theirs.

Hebrews 13:1-2: Let brotherly love continue. Don't neglect to show hospitality, for by doing this some have welcomed angels as guests without knowing it. (HCS)

Chapter III

DEATH OF THE SOUL
(Loss of the Star Dust)

1 Samuel 2:6: The Lord brings death and gives life; He sends some to Sheol, and He raises others up. (HCS)

Romans 5:14: Nevertheless, death reigned from Adam to Moses, even over those who did not sin in the likeness of Adam's transgression. He is the prototype of the Coming One. (HCS)

Interpretation of Romans 5:14: Death has engulfed the human Soul since the introduction of the industries connected to the Rod of Asclepius Symbol. Soul death will continue up to the point when humanity steps out of Egypt (Moses), representative of moving away from the systems of industries in the world today that enslave. There are certain individuals that have advanced to Heaven during this period of time. There are specifications that apply here.

Revelation 7:4 should be considered. "And I heard the number of those who were sealed: 144,000 sealed from every tribe of the Israelites:" (HCS)

There has been a dangerous lack of proper education about what the Soul is and how it functions. Many persons have died an eternal death because of the unseen influence modern day healthcare, and other sources, can and does have on the Soul. The Energy that comes from the cosmos and takes up residence in the blood cells is what the Soul is comprised of, the Star Dust. Modern day medical imaging and treatments, toxins and chemicals interfere with the health of the Star Dust. Anything that influences the blood also influences the Soul.

There are two types of death, death of the physical body and death of the Soul.

Soul/Star Dust status:
1) A person is born with an elevated level of Star Dust;
2) A person is born with a minimal level of Star Dust;
3) A person is born with no Star Dust and is simply a material mortal being.

Level 1: Jesus is an example of one born on earth yet had an elevated level of Star Dust upon arrival. His life story reflects how that Star Dust level can increase or decrease given circumstances, and how when persistence and tenacity is in place obstacles can be overcome and you have the opportunity to return "Home" as an eternal being via the volume and quality of Star Dust. Star Dust is the Soul, the collective Energy received by humans from the cosmos.

Level 2: I believe many people are born with a level of Star Dust but not necessarily an abundance given the level of toxicity prior generations have been exposed to. Star Dust activation occurs during the sixth month of gestation in connection with specific phases of the moon and/or with a lot of specifics attached. Gender is also determined by the phase of the moon. Life experiences and choices can and often do deplete the Star Dust level and depending upon where that level is upon the death of the person whether they will graduate to an eternal being or whether their Soul simply does not have enough Star Dust to keep them alive after departure from the physical body and the Soul fades away.

Prior to what is described as "the Day of the Lord" in Scripture some Souls would progress to a place called Purgatory to sleep or rest until an appointed time. The Soul was without sufficient Star Dust to advance to Heaven or to become eternal at the time of death so the Soul was gathered into a resting place. I call this place the Spa, a place where refreshment is in order. The events surrounding the "Day of the Lord" will bring about two things: 1) those who have been in Purgatory resting will advance on to their eternal Home/Heaven; 2) at a given point after the Day of the Lord, each individual living person will be responsible for maintaining the level of Star Dust required to advance to "eternal," leaving one to conclude that Purgatory will no longer be in use. You either graduate to eternal, or not. There is no longer a resting place.

As time progresses and people receive and maintain a healthy level of Star Dust, the frequencies generated by the Star Dust can be used to assist others. This idea runs parallel with the stories of Jesus healing the sick. There is an activity that will begin to occur in a form of cellular communication between one person and another. This can be compared to how your cell phone works. The contacts that you have stored in your cell phone will be the ones you most often share communication with. I bring up this scenario because it is this cellular communication that will advance the life of the Soul and eliminate the need for Purgatory.

Galatians 6:1-5: Brothers, if someone is caught in any wrongdoing, you who are spiritual should restore such a person with a gentle spirit, watching out for yourselves so you also won't be tempted. (This is speaking of a transfer of "sin" frequencies within the cells from one person to another. A person with healthy Star Dust (one who has a gift of being a "Healer") can assist one who is ill but the Healer must use caution in order to avoid the illness transferring to him/her.) *v. 2: Carry one another's burdens; in this way you will fulfill the law of Christ.* (The term "Christ" is indicative of a status in the blood. This verse is speaking of the communication between one person's blood and another's.) *v. 3: For if anyone considers himself to be something when he is nothing, he deceives himself.* (This is speaking of an individual being certain there is sufficient Star Dust to eliminate his/her personal sin or sickness when there isn't.) *v. 4: But each person should examine his own work, and then he will have a reason for boasting in himself alone, and not in respect to someone else.* (This is speaking about building Star Dust up to the point you can maintain yourself vs. having to rely on others to assist you in overcoming or warding off a physical affliction.) *v. 5: For each person will have to carry his own load.* (Eventually, each person is going to need to know how to receive and maintain the Star Dust level it takes to remain healthy and become eternal.) These verses describe the practices of the Wise Men and Wise Women (Healers) of Ancient times.

Level 3: The third situation is when a person is born simply mortal. They can live life here on earth but the blood lacks the elements necessary to connect the person to the cosmic Energy that deposits the Star Dust into the cells. At the time of physical death there is no Soul that would transcend.

Influence of Vibration

There are mysterious, magical, magnetic elements that exist in the atmosphere and they can be influenced by the presence of vibration. Vibrations are a result of many things, including movement, walking, vehicles, and vocals, speaking or singing. Every person, plant, animal, color, and so on came into existence as a result of collective vibrations. Genesis 1:3: Then God said (or spoke) indicative of vibration being the initiator of creation.

Imagine a magnetic field that joins with vibrations and suspends in and moves through airspace that is void of objects, such as open fields, or space in the sky. This may be what a Dust/Dirt Devil seen moving through a field is comprised of. Once these collective vibrations intersect with a material item, a reaction occurs. The cluster of magnetic particles, enhanced by vibration produce what I call Charged Clouds and these Charged Clouds can influence weather patterns or intensity, the physical body and so on. Think of this like a vapor cloud, an influence that is there yet not seen. Ever felt as though you were swimming upstream just to complete a daily task? There may be a Charged Cloud to blame.

When a Charged Cloud becomes overloaded with or encounters a combination of vibrations at some point those Charged Clouds will manifest an event. Example: August of 2023 Taylor Swift event at SoFi Stadium in Los Angeles created seismic activity equivalent to a 2.0 magnitude earthquake. Music pushed through amplifiers and speakers have a huge impact on our surroundings and our physical bodies through the production of static electricity. This is one way the electrical charge within the cells (Star Dust) is compromised, through excessive levels of static electricity and vibration.

Knowledge with respect to the impact vibrations can have on the body is lacking. Vibrations record in the cells and will later reveal themselves in symptoms or characteristics of descendants. An interesting example of this is a young man I knew, I will call him Pete, at times would enter a room with a sort of rhythmic bounce style dance similar to maybe a break dance. The episode would be brief and more of a silly expression of excess energy. I often wondered where these dances came from, why would someone suddenly have an urge to wiggle in this way when no music was playing and the atmosphere was not inviting for such displays. Later in years I would learn that Pete's mother would frequent dance clubs in her youth. This fact put the pieces of the mystery together. The vibrations from the music played at the dance club were recorded in Pete's mother's cells and transferred to Pete at some point during pregnancy. What Pete was displaying was a reenactment of the dancing to the music done by his mother in prior years. This may also explain why Pete would often wake quite early in the morning. Going to sleep at night was not a problem but staying asleep was problematic for him and waking at 3:00, 4:00 or 5:00 in the morning was common. The secret lives of ancestors will come to the surface at some point!

A similar type action/reaction occurs in the body when the electrical charge in the cells becomes overloaded with toxins, chemicals, food preservatives, and so forth, setting the stage for an explosive event – disease erupts. The healthy or balanced vibration that sustains the electrical charge experiences a change.

Things absorbed through the skin or ingested can simply pass through the body. It's the essence (vibration) those things leave behind while passing through the body that create a physical response, good, bad or indifferent. Yes, the body is built to filter out the material objects encountered, it is the essence of those things that become stuck in the body due to the lost art of cleansing methods that can result in a destructive internal fire.

Matthew 15:16-17: Are even you still lacking in understanding? He asked. Don't you realize that whatever goes into the mouth passes into the stomach and is eliminated? (HCS)

Exposure to toxins, noise and involvement in numerous worldly traditions will have a negative influence on the Star Dust. The Charged Clouds that develop through activities will influence the Star Dust as well. A good example of activities that produce Charged Clouds is traditional holiday celebrations and funerals.

Why is this important and what does it have to do with cancers and disease?

As previously stated, cancer is a collective disease. The more a person is exposed to harmful environments, toxins and so on, the greater the chances are for cancer to come forth. Cancer is the evidence of overload of exposure.

Soul Banking

Think of the Soul like a bank account that receives deposits and transactions of debits. A person obviously wants an account that reflects a level of comfort or wealth and this same concept works with the Soul. A wealthy

Soul account is a healthy Soul. When Scripture references an inheritance it is speaking of the value held within the Soul at the time of a person's departure from earth. If a person dies with a wealthy Soul account their heirs will receive a deposit. A similar concept applies with bankrupt Souls. When a person with a bankrupt Soul dies leaving debts unpaid, the balance due gets transferred to the heirs. Flipping the Ancient "as above, so below" concept around, one could say "what goes on down here is reflective of how things work up (or out) there." Disease lurks between the measure of the average Soul account and a bankrupt Soul account. Encountering a Charged Cloud can debit a Soul account.

A downward progression of the Soul will cease once a specific status is reached. You can think of this like graduating from college, once you have passed through the various stages and tests your knowledge is secured. Steady income through the profession in response to the education begins. You have the ability to keep the bills paid with income leftover. Tossing aside what has been learned and becoming lazy is not an option in order to avoid a sickened Soul or depleted Star Dust.

What is the root issue to the death of the Soul?

I don't hold the answers for the entire circumference of this question. I believe there is more than one root to the issue and the three main roots appear to have numerous offshoots. 1) Food/Diet; 2) Misuse of Symbols and Misappropriation of Symbolic Acts; 3) Worldly Systems.

It is becoming more and more clear that in some respects humans have brewed up their own systems and standards that have lead to their demise. A manmade form of booby trap is continually expanding.

The general public has been informed by "those who test it and inspect it" that products are safe to use or consume prior to their availability. Tests have been had and the stamp of approval applied. No one admits to being responsible for any resulting damage or harm yet people have been handed products and told they are safe to use only to be led along a road that results in a self-induced form of suicide. The medical industry doesn't take responsibility, nor does the pharmaceutical industry, the food industry, the electronic industry, the dental industry, the environmental and safety industry, and so forth. Each throws up their hands with a shout of, "it's not my fault!" A shadow of guilt is present upon them all. One stand-alone product from any one industry likely would not cause insurmountable health issues but add one to the other, and another, and another and you have an overload of stress on the body. The stage becomes set for the potential loss of the Soul.

Proverbs 21:6: Making a fortune through a lying tongue is a vanishing mist, a pursuit of death. (HCS)

Chapter IV

LANGUAGE OF THE COSMOS
Symbols and Symbolic Acts

Symbols hold a value all their own. For thousands of years Symbols were a means of communication, long before numerals and alphabet. What is a Symbol?

Symbol: Something that represents something else by association, resemblance, or convention, especially a material object used to represent something invisible; an instance that typifies a broader pattern or situation.

A contributor to the downfall in the quality of life for humans and for the earth and all that is within it is the misunderstanding or lack of understanding with respect to Symbols. Symbols will initiate an energetic response from the cosmos.

The following paragraphs contain past and current situations that have created a Symbolic value that has been received and transcribed by the Energies in the cosmos/Heavens. Think of the entire circumference of the cosmos as a recording station. The collective Symbolic energies in the cosmos are eventually transmitted to the earth in forms of beneficial or harmful situations that are encouraged by the Symbolic Energies received. (As above, so below.) It is as though the Symbol itself or the Symbolic Act(s) on earth, particularly when a person in a position of power or authority is involved, ascend to the cosmos by a means of vibration. Those vibrations are collected and form a good or bad invisible force that descends back to the earth, influencing the persons or location from which the originating Symbolic Act took place. Because the returned communication coming to the earth is of an invisible electrical influence, that communication will influence a human on a cellular level. A good visual for this concept is the Native American Rain Dance. A series of motions that create vibrations that ascend to the cosmos/Heavens and eventually produce a response, hopefully in the form of moisture. Also, think of this like cell phone communication. Someone leaves a message on your cell phone then you retrieve the message and are influenced in some manner by that message. Symbols and Symbolic Acts work in a like manner. Have you ever heard the phrase "what goes around comes around?" Same concept. The initiating Symbolic Act or display of a Symbol will bring the unseen influence of such Symbol/Act full circle causing a form of repeated circumstance(s).

The lost art of Symbolic representation through traditions and daily activity must be recaptured. The Heavens respond to Symbols and Symbolic Acts. It is the language used and understood in that realm. Every act we involve ourselves in has a Symbolic value. Symbols have great impact on an atmosphere. Symbols can be an actual material object such as Stonehenge, a cross or even sundials. A Symbolic Act read by the cosmos will take on the form of an action, something acted out throughout a day such as doing the laundry or going to the bank. Certain Symbols or Symbolic Acts relay a message of benefit and some relay a message of demise. This language and its impact on daily life is a key component in the not so merry Merry-Go-Round Humanity appears to be on.

The signal given off by a Symbol catches in the airwaves and showers down to those within reach or connected to that particular Symbol. Another way to look at the resulting energies from Symbols is with the Charged Cloud analogy. <u>Example of a result from a Symbolic Act</u>: When a person lives in or spends many hours while working in a tall building the cosmic signals sent to that person relay a message to the cells of height, to be tall; a signal to reach for the clouds or climb higher. As generations progress, genetics will manifest by producing individuals connected to the person who spent time in a tall building, who are tall. The Symbol of tall buildings gave rise to the incident of tall descendants.

Influence of a Symbol: A cross is a very popular Symbol. Crosses decorate many hillsides, hospital reception spaces, churches and homes. Unknown to many is a cross in the form of the standard Christian Cross actually represents suffering and death. This representation is evident in the story of the Crucifixion.

<u>Deuteronomy 21:22-23</u>: If anyone is found guilty of an offense deserving the death penalty and is executed, and you hang his body on a tree, you are not to leave his corpse on the tree overnight but are to bury him that day, for anyone hung on a tree is under God's curse. You must not defile the land the Lord you God is giving you as an inheritance. (HCS) (Land is a reference to lifestyle.)

<u>Galatians 3:13</u>: Christ has redeemed us from the curse of the law by becoming a curse for us, because it is written:

Everyone who is hung on a tree is cursed. (HCS) (The term "Christ" represents a status of the blood.)

Symbolic Power of Those in Authority

Actions displayed by persons in a position of authority have a Symbolic value that can influence all residing within their reigning sphere. A Mayor has a sphere within the boundaries of his/her city, and so forth through the channels of governing positions. An Example of Symbolic Act Influence: If the Mayor of a city is a thief, there is an unseen essence of attraction for thieves to want to frequent, reside in or that do reside in the city the Mayor Thief is in position over. The essence of "being a thief" can remain within that city even after the term of Mayor Thief comes to an end. It is as though the activity of thievery is stuck in the atmosphere.

This concept is true for all levels of governing positions and persons with a legal authority. The Symbolic lifestyle of each person in a ruling position has a huge unseen influence on those under their particular ruling authority.

I am far from being a politician and have never cared much for politics. With the wisdom I have gained about Symbols and Symbolic Acts and how they influence everything in the "unseen," I realize that the dishonest mud flinging characteristics stamped throughout politics and shouted over airwaves in what is called political speeches and campaigns is contributing to the deterioration of the United States and the people who reside within its borders. The atmosphere becomes overloaded with the essence of the governing official's characteristics that have been or are on display. Disagreements or contentious conversations should be had in private behind professional closed doors not broadcast through tabloids or public electronic broadcasting systems.

Leaders who participate in activities that are far from professional and take steps to cover up their dealings are depositing corruption into the airwaves that create an atmosphere that can, and will eventually, take on a similar manifestation in either other persons or businesses. These are the classifications of persons who are leading this nation and their actions speak volumes for the nation as a whole. This is a good place to insert: What Goes Around Comes Around.

I am certain many teachers in our government controlled schools would confess to the often unruly youth within their classrooms where back talking, name calling and unacceptable conversations brew. Highways (government owned property) are full of drivers who have unruly driving habits and have no problem displaying their personal dislike for someone driving the speed limit. These situations are manifestations of the actions taken by leaders sprinkled through this nation. Leaders plant the seeds for these characteristics.

A detailed review of historical events that have preceded the current generations reveals some interesting initiations of how humanity stepped onto this endless cycle of sickness and disease, among other things. For 248 years and counting the United States has experienced levels of decline and decay initiated by an act of rebellion that led to separation. Fourth of July celebrations symbolically shout to the cosmos that Americans are satisfied with separation, a form of death in relationships.

A case of exaggerated emotional flare-ups that resulted in the separation of the United Colonies from her mate, the British Empire, radiates a message of division within the now United States of America. The emotions from the events that led to the preparation and signing of the Declaration of Independence remain in the atmosphere. The life of independence resounds thousands of times each year throughout the USA, manifesting in the forms of household divorce, family relationship breakups, children disowning parents and visa versa, business relationships dissolving, and so forth. This display of independence through a document signed by those in official positions not only tears the family unit apart but also separates nations resulting in battlefields that take lives.

How is the cyclical separation problem solved?

European ancestral roots herald for many Americans, the homeland of those who preceded many of us. The uniting of the United States of America with the Crown of England would bring a sense of security to this nation, a union, rather than the lost and wondering vagabond she has been. It is time to see the truth and pay reverence to the Source that controls all life and death and make peace with our Mother Country, England.

Think this theory holds no ground? Turn back to the page that lists the percentages of prescription drugs consumed by adults in the U.S. vs. the percentage of prescription drugs consumed by those in the U.K. before you decide. It is the unseen fragrance of historical events that can build into various forms of destruction.

It is time to make amends. Prince Harry, I welcome you and your family to the United States and pray that your residing in the United States is a Symbolic Act of the Crown being legally joined to the United States once again.

For peace to be had, the United States of America must take steps to become the United Colonies once again, healing the cycle of decay, death, and deterioration. If you have ever wondered why the death rate is increasing, what I have just explained may be a contributing factor because the symbolism of death has been stamped all across America through the sands of time with an initiation point being what is called The Declaration of Independence. What was documented and signed holds great impact and declaring a country to be separated from Royalty and the Crown has done more harm than what anyone will likely ever understand.

Stuck in a Death Sentence

Again, when an individual in a position of governing authority, say a King, President or appointed religious authority, takes action or executes a legal document it becomes recorded in the cosmic atmosphere, in the airwaves. Example: executing an order and relative action taken that initiates a death sentence.

In the 1500s authorities from various positions and status prepared and executed a document ordering the death of those who lived as or displayed activities of what has received the title of "Witch." This action planted a seed in the cosmos that all people who have a particular blood code connected to "Witch" should be put to death in some form or fashion. This equates to any descendant of those the Order for Death influenced receiving the same or similar sentence over their life. The blood is what transmits signals that attract the attention of the cosmos.

Even though we are hundreds of years down the road from the origination of the Order executed, the record still remains in the cosmos as though it was signed yesterday. Anyone with a percentage of DNA that connects them to the persons ordered to be put to death will likely encounter various challenges throughout their lifetime that are an attempt to take their life; life appears to work against them. My "Journey of a Life Time" illustrates a perfect example of this. Whether those attempts are in the form of accidents or disease, the cosmos is responding to the Order it received many years prior. To reverse this cosmic death sentence, a person in a position of power must override the original Order(s).

Proverbs 20:2: A king's terrible wrath is like the roaring of a lion; anyone who provokes him endangers himself. (HCS)

Symbolic Influence of Holidays and Special Events

Mark 7:8-9: Disregarding the command of God, you keep the tradition of men. He also said to them, you completely invalidate God's command in order to maintain your tradition! (HCS)

There is no logical or scientific explanation for the situations presented. When a person becomes familiar with how Energy reacts to a given movement or process, what is being described becomes easier to follow. The impact from improper celebrations will be on the interior of the body not necessarily being immediately evident.

Americanized holidays are, at times, altered reflections of spiritual concepts, modified in ways that damage rather than benefit. Cosmic activity responds to Symbols and those Symbols will draw a good or bad response dependant upon what the Symbol means and how it is being used. The atmosphere created by inappropriate (according to Spirit standards and laws) holiday celebrations will deplete or even damage the Soul. The Star Dust suffers an impact. The acts of celebrations at the incorrect time or place, some according to the phase of the moon, can and in some cases will, alter the elements of the blood.

Participation in some traditional Americanized holidays can result in a harmful impact on the brain, afflicting the memory. Some holiday celebrations afflict the chromosomes, and some can stir up angry, harmful Energy in an atmosphere. These gatherings that are contrary to the laws of nature and the laws of the cosmos also contribute to the emotional disturbances sometimes displayed at family gatherings.

Various medical conditions can result from participation in incorrect holiday celebrations. What seems to be the common denominator is food of varying types being combined and consumed in the same meal minus the proper practices to aid in removal all of the interior chaos created by those foods.

Amos 8:10: I will turn your feasts into mourning and all your songs into lamentation; I will cause everyone to wear sackcloth and every head to be shaved. I will make that grief like mourning for an only son and its outcome like a bitter day. (HCS)

Reference to a shaved head is Symbolic of a bald head, whether a result of chemotherapy or genetics. In other words, a bald head can be a result of feasting at times that are contrary to the laws of nature.

Thanksgiving feasts have produced genetics for being tired or lazy. How? By eating turkey that contains tryptophan on a date and/or at a time of day that meat or feasting is not to be had. Meat is to be eaten at twilight and prepared in a specific manner and consumed only when wearing specific attire. The steps to remove the damaging influence of meat were lost long ago so the energetic influence became stuck in the blood/DNA. Could Dementia or even Alzheimer's be in this category as well? See, Exodus, Chapter 16.

A holiday many relate to is Christmas. Christmas trees, usually of an Evergreen, have roots in Pagan history. According to history, a number of Pagan authorities converted to Christianity, such as the Viking leader Rollo. The conversions appear to have been an effort to gain access to or take control over land and/or the people within it. The more you delve into the history of these types of activities that took place, the more it becomes clear that Pagan roots found their way in the door of Christianity and produced a mixed breed.

The popular Christmas color red is Symbolic of the blood. Colors coupled with red will have an influence on the blood. Black with red would give off a signal of darkness; white with red would give off a signal of washing things out, a fading. Green with red has a significant influence and should not be worn or displayed together. What about giving or receiving gifts? There are many Scriptures on gifts. The extent of influence on these subjects will need to be explored at a later time. How many other holiday traditions could be damaging to the Soul?

Many roots of Easter come from Pagan traditions: Ham, bunnies and colored eggs, to name a few. CreationCalendar.com shared an interesting article on the history and influence of Easter in March 2024. Taking a few moments to look up the article would cast light on the subject for the reader.

Birthday celebrations are another tradition that can afflict the Soul. Again, we are untangling the mysteries of Symbols. Candle lighting holds significance as does eating (white) cake. The symbolism of fire speaks of offerings being sent up to the Heavens and when displayed improperly creates a mockery of the original intention thereof. The cosmic atmosphere reads the candle fire within its own language, not how we think of it, as a sign to mark years of age. Taking a form of fire and placing it upon a cake has a level of impact energetically that is yet to be fully grasped.

No fire is to be present on a Sabbath day. (Exodus 16:23) Not only the act of preparing foods is to be eliminated on a Sabbath but also there are repeated references to the source used to cook the food, being fire for roasting or boiling that should be avoided on a Sabbath. How many birthday celebrations, or even weddings, with candles have taken place on a Sabbath (Saturday)? Too many to count.

Some myths reference cake as being a "food of the gods," which would translate to mean cake is only for a person who has achieved a specific blood chemistry, or has sin-free or infection-free blood; one who has escaped the afflictions and now qualifies for becoming/or is eternal.

Genesis 40:20: On the third day, which was Pharaoh's birthday, he gave a feast for all his servants. He lifted up the heads of the chief cupbearer and the chief baker. (HCS) (emphasis added)

Interpretation of Genesis 40:20: A power (Pharaoh) exists within birthday celebrations particularly those held on the "third day" that afflict the head; drinking (cupbearer) and eating (baker connects to pastries or cakes) are involved. With the Gregorian calendaring system, many today do not know when the "third day" takes place. All fingers pointing to some form of cosmic activity that takes place that will influence the brain/head.

Job 1:18-19: He was still speaking when another messenger came and reported: "Your sons and daughters were eating and drinking wine in their oldest brother's house. Suddenly a powerful wind swept in from the desert and struck the four corners of the house. It collapsed on the young people so that they died, and I alone have escaped to tell you!" (HCS)

Interpretation of Job 1:18-19: Birthday gathering brewed up adversity and manifested in the form of a wind resulting in demise by afflicting the respiratory system. Wind translates to something that comes against you; in Vedic Hymns wind represents the breath. Some translations of Scripture replace the reference of birthday with banquet. A birthday with a celebration that involves eating and drinking wine. In this instance wine refers to the blood. There is a deadly influence on the condition of the blood. Reference to oldest brother indicates an age related gathering, most commonly a birthday, otherwise there would be no need to reference the age. The house in this case represents a specific group of persons with a common belief or tradition; in all directions means around the globe (four corners). Young people that died references Soul death; harm comes to the Soul, which is comprised of the blood. Again, the reference to the age as "young" reflects a death not relative to the physical body, which normally dies at an old age.

What about Mother's Day or other recognition days? Here's something to consider:

Why did Jesus refer to his mother as "woman," both at the cross and at the wedding feast? By this time in the life of Jesus He was an adult, capable of conducting His life business and decisions. Could these instances of referring to His mother as "woman" be telling us that the duties of a mother are limited to the time of conception to adulthood, whatever age that may be given the culture you reside in, say 15-18 years old. After a child reaches adulthood they no longer need "mother"; by this time a son/daughter should be well trained in worldly decision making, and so forth. The same goes for fathering; there is a limited window for fathering/mothering services outside of a special needs situation.

It appears that the Greeting Card industry has the world by the tail, once again lining their pockets on holidays or recognition days that are wholly man's idea.

Funerals

There are specific protocols for burying a corpse in order to avoid the display of a Symbolic signal to the atmosphere that those participating in honoring the deceased want to receive a form of death. It's one thing to honor a deceased or their family, it's another issue to endanger your own health in the process. Delivering a corpse into a church sanctuary for a funeral service is quite harmful to the atmosphere people are sitting in. A sanctuary is Symbolic of the inner most being of the human body, a private space. Whatever is in a church sanctuary will produce in a similar manner within the interior of the human body. This falls under the category of "Law of Attraction."

A foundational root of the Epstein Barr Virus originates from the exact environment described, death within a sanctuary. EBV is a very destructive virus causing sore throat, swollen glands, overloaded lymph, fever, extreme fatigue, and eventually can lead to cancer. Sounds like a death sentence to me.

A separate establishment should house the corpse during all funeral related activities and transported from that establishment to the burial site, never entering a sanctuary. If you have ever wondered why Jesus said "let the dead bury the dead," this is why. Those who have an increased level of Star Dust will suffer a loss of that Star Dust by being in the situations just described. Those who have no Star Dust are those Jesus spoke of as "the dead" who would bury the corpse.

Matthew 8:21-22: "Lord," another of His disciples said, "first let me go bury my father." But Jesus told him, "Follow Me, and let the dead bury their own dead." (HCS)

Not only are there harmful Charged Clouds that are produced when a corpse is taken into the sanctuary of a church, but eating while grieving has consequences as well. King David declared an oath stating:

2 Samuel 3:32-35: When they buried Abner in Hebron, the king wept aloud at Abner's tomb. All the people wept, and the king sang a lament for Abner: Should Abner die as a fool dies? Your hands were not bound, your feet not placed in bronze shackles. You fell like one who falls victim to criminals. All the people wept over him even more. Then they came to urge David to eat bread while it was still day, but David took an oath: **"May God punish me and do so severely if I taste bread or anything else before sunset!"** *(HCS)* (emphasis added)

When grieving, a person must wait until after sunset to partake of food in order to avoid a setback in their health or depletion of Star Dust. The chemical reaction between the grieving process and foods create a toxic environment for the body.

Flower blooms will influence the Star Dust levels as well. Flowers have their own energies and can be thought of like static electricity that will stick to you, interfering with the electrical charge within you. Flower buds and blooms also have a Symbolic value of being temporary; those that fade away. Funerals are to be celebrated with lights, indicative of the light within the Soul, not flowers.

Any single exposure to these situations is likely not Soul-life threatening. It is when they continue to add up with no forms of replenishment for the Soul in place that the Soul becomes threatened.

Many activities and substances encountered on a daily basis in this day and time cause a level of damage to the Soul. Understanding the language of the cosmos, which consists of Symbols, has been lost. Participating in actions relative to many traditional holidays has turned an intended joyful celebration into a disaster simply because the Symbols displayed draw an unwanted form of cosmic electricity or prevents an opportunity to receive a cosmic recharge for the Soul. You get what you ask for.

Chapter V

SILENT KILLERS

Chemistry and Buffet Style Eating

The physical body has become a chemistry project gone-wrong. The buffet style eating coupled with non-stop electro-magnetic exposure and toxic compounds that are in food, water, scented candles, toiletries, cleaning agents, and lush green grass, the chemical structures within the body have become a mess. I confess to have never taken a chemistry class nor had any success at reading and deciphering a chemical equation. The conclusions presented are a product of observation and personal experience, coupled with common sense.

The Standard American Diet packs a body with various categories of food, flavors and colors many times on any one day. Those foods, coupled with acidic coffees, teas or other acidic drinks, sometimes with carbonation, and excess water intake make their way through the body to the stomach for processing. The eating and digestion process is taking place in an environment of approximately 98 degrees with no means of appropriate ventilation for the level of gases being produced by the feast of food just eaten. Here's where the belches and well, let's call it flatulence, all of which are chalked up as "normal" come into play. When the mix-match of food intake is done day after day and let's throw in a digestive upset or backup in the drain pipes (intestines) the contents consumed sit additional hours releasing gases. The production of gases begins to have an influence on organs and systems in the body. Think of it like making fermented foods. I attempted to make fermented cabbage once by packing a quart jar full of chopped cabbage, threw in a few spices and other ingredients the recipe called for, screwed the lid on and placed it in the refrigerator, a much cooler environment than the temperature inside the body. After a few days the entire refrigerator smelled of a putrid gas. Needless to say, the fermenting project went into the trash. Take this visual and apply it to the body; add the increase in consumption of water (man's idea), to the fermenting food in the digestive tract, the heat that is accumulating in the body due to the natural order of body temperature, and the gases being produced and we can now throw in condensation. Condensation is a breeding ground for bacteria. Ever wonder why your neighbor has that distended pregnancy looking belly?

If the majority of a diet consists of a broad variety of foods that produce an internal heat (such as hot peppers, spicy foods or boiled soups) and that food along with acidic, carbonated or alcohol based drinks brewed together and cause an internal environment of excessive chemical reactions that form gases, the house (body) will eventually catch fire and burn down! The body has become a walking fire hazard.

Baker's yeast produces a chemical reaction and is frequently mentioned in Scripture. With yeast being a common topic in Scripture and certainly a commonly consumed product, it would make sense that a concern for contamination of the blood could be had. I suggest that there are unidentified microbial substances that are present in yeast that result in sepsis when proper eating and cleansing protocols are lacking. This brings up the question of whether brewer's yeast would have a same or similar contaminating influence. Evidence of a microbial infection in the blood is thin or thinning hair.

Leviticus 2:11: No grain offering that you present to the Lord is to be made with yeast, for you are not to burn any yeast or honey as a fire offering to the Lord. (HCS)

The Old Testament Scriptures that speak of presenting an offering are referring to a process that takes place inside the body, a chemical reaction or essence from the particular item being consumed.

1 Corinthians 5:6-8: Your boasting is not good. Don't you know that a little yeast permeates the whole batch of dough? Clean out the old yeast so that you may be a new batch. You are indeed unleavened for Christ our Passover has been sacrificed. Therefore, let us observe the feast, not with old yeast or with the yeast of malice and evil but with the unleavened bread of sincerity and truth. (HCS)

It only takes a small amount of yeast to influence the whole body, specifically the blood. In order to reach the status of Christ (more details on this in my book From Antichrist to I AM published 2022), the blood must be clean and that includes having no contaminates, particularly those that originate from yeast. Reference to Passover is speaking of decay and disease not coming to you because there is no "yeast" (microbial) to be found in you.

There is an unidentified microbial infection that originates from yeast and has a harmful, potentially deadly influence on the blood and ultimately the Soul. According to Leviticus 2:11, yeast and honey should not be consumed together and/or at a specified time. This gives rise to the question if yeast has the potential to elevate or alter bacteria that are naturally present in honey. How many other food items could yeast have a negative influence on? Or, how many food items are potentially damaging given the phase of the moon?

Looking at a Periodic Table of Elements there are quite a few chemical elements, evidence of many components being involved. One answer to disease lies in the chemical makeup of the blood to which no sufficient chemical equation exists for interpreting what the blood is saying, otherwise many health mysteries would have previously been solved.

Previously established tables and formulas used today in classrooms and laboratories are lacking and should be tossed out. It is apparent, particularly within the medical industry, that the previously generated and established tables and formulas contain flaws that result in incomplete or incorrect conclusions. A new standard must be created to capture the truth of events taking place within the body, specifically the blood.

It would be an added benefit for all of the "reference ranges" set in blood analysis to be re-evaluated, expanded and new ranges established. Many times over I've heard from people that state how a cancer or other life threatening condition was not evident to their physician until late stages of the disease. More imaging is not the answer. A more in depth blood analysis is necessary to hear what the blood is saying. In my case, by the time any WBC count would have exceeded the current standard reference range, the train would have already been wrecked and full recovery unreachable. When a disease becomes active and is reflected through a blood analysis, why is it that the blood itself is not sufficiently treated, or treated at all? Instead, treatments are given to control or ease the symptom that is being produced by an affliction to the blood, likely stemming from an infection of a bacterial nature. Appears the prescribed remedy for the disease is incomplete. A question would be, can infections create or attract a static electricity that eventually gives rise to cancer?

Nutrients

Are the nutritional combinations that fall under a standardized acceptance contributing to the harmful influence the cells encounter when exposure to specific substances or environments is had? The accepted nutritional standards and guidelines for daily nutritional intake were established several years ago with the government producing guidelines between 1970-1980s. By this point in time, much of the human blood was already on a highway to contamination or alteration, resulting in test conclusions that were used to set such standards likely being flawed. When the baseline is contaminated, the results will be negatively influenced.

Even though my diet consisted of organic, fresh foods, and fast foods had not been on my plate for several years, I had a bacterial infection that had developed in my blood, never identified by an M.D., nor even considered. Energy testing via a computer repeatedly sounded alarms for "bacteria" but figuring out where it was seemed nearly impossible.

When the health setback I experienced in October of 2020 occurred, my spine at C5, C6, and C7 was swollen and looked like golf balls. This was likely, never proven, a parking place for the infection. This bacteria had reached my brain and resulted in periodic stabbing pains on the top of my head when I would wake in the morning, random tooth pain, and the bacteria eventually worked its way through a top molar to the point a root canal was necessary and a post implanted due to the level of decay that had taken place from the root down through the tooth. How is this type of bacteria not detectible by the medical industry? Someone, anyone? This screams the fact that research is lacking and science and the medical industry have a long way to go in order to capture and treat infections, or the chemical combinations contributing to infection, that are more common than believed.

Personally, I believe it was the bacteria driving me to a leukemia diagnosis that the genetic panel revealed I had a double mutation for. I lost an Aunt in 2019 that had leukemia giving rise to the fact leukemia was in the family genetics. Had I not taken steps on my own to remedy the issue, my address would currently be engraved upon a headstone.

Static Electricity

Luke 21:26: People will faint from fear and expectation of the things that are coming on the world, because the celestial powers will be shaken. Then they will see the Son of Man coming in a cloud with power and great glory. (HCS) (emphasis added)

What is static electricity? Two brief definitions: Static electricity is the result of an imbalance between negative and positive charges; a stationary electric charge typically produced by friction.

Humans are not alone in the negative/positive electrical charge disturbance, the earth herself is out of balance in her negative/positive electrical charge. It is as though the earth has become a suspended ball of static electricity. Ever feel as though everything you touch gives off an electric shock? I have noticed an increase of a general tiredness just from being outdoors. Could all this imbalance in electrical charge be a result of humans not being in what I call "the Adam Status" to assist in the proper balance of electrical charge? Or is it the over production of toxic compounds that are to blame? Likely it is a combination of both of these situations.

Could static electricity in the atmosphere be an answer to heart attacks? The heart is run by electricity so it would make sense that inference in its rhythm would come from an opposing electrical source. Add a microbial infection that is in the blood and the electrical function in the body becomes stressed.

Plastics can create a disaster all their own. Plastic can migrate to the brain and interfere with the electrical activity in the brain resulting in disturbances. Plastics also contribute to the accumulation of static electricity, as does stainless steel appliances that decorate many homes today. Ever notice how much dust your stainless steel appliances attract? This static electricity related dance is likely a contributor to electric disruption within the earth, and the body and contributes to a body not having the proper ability to heal itself, presenting a grand opportunity for cancers and other disease.

For those familiar with metaphors, each part of the home is representative of a collective group of persons and the influence each part of that home plays in the dance we call life. Appliances all have their reflective influence, as does furniture, plumbing fixtures, and so forth. For those who can follow me, let's take this a little further. If a refrigerator represents the cooling components within the body with respect to food consumption and digestion, and the actual refrigerator in a home is producing an imbalance in the negative/positive charge as stainless steel does, would that Symbolic manifestation result in a physical affliction with respect to cooling the body as it takes in food? Are we telling the cosmic atmosphere that we wish to have an imbalance in the negative/positive charge within our body resulting in a disturbance of the cooling process when we eat our food? What a mess! All at the hands of mankind and innovative ideas.

There is some form of fanciful activity going on inside the body that Scientists, Researchers or Chemists have yet to discover or they are not sharing what they know with the medical industry and the public. If they are at a loss, I point in the direction of chemical imbalances that result in harmful gas production, a static electricity component and a more in depth research on microbial in yeast.

Industries that produce chemical based products that alone have their own form of static electricity need more stringent regulations and restrictions. Mounds upon mounds of plastic products, synthetics and other static producing items are a contributing factor to the over abundance of static electricity influencing us all, including the earth.

With the earth having an unusual level of static electricity, if in doubt I direct attention to the amount of lightning storms seen in many areas over the past few years, what is this radiating static electricity doing to the human body even through simple outdoor exposure? For the past several years when I attempt an outdoor time of walking or hiking my leg muscles would become heavy, painful and feel as though they were in knots. What is influencing the leg muscles in this way? Could it be an imbalance in the negative/positive charge in the soil or the air? I am not a weakling and have actually had physicians ask what type of exercise I do because my blood analysis would reflect that I was regularly exercising. To their surprise I would inform them that I do not regularly exercise but I do remain active.

The improper eating and drinking habits coupled with excessive exposure to electro-magnetic fields and static electricity has the makings of a death trap. The question is how do you undo all of the eating habits, comforts and traditions people have lived by for hundreds of years? Harder still is getting people to change their lifestyle, traditions and customs. The best remedy: Inform, and allow for personal choice.

Identification

There must be an underlying, unidentified chemical or electrical component in the human blood that has yet to be discovered and it has nothing to do with the blood types of A, O, B, AB. Once this unidentified component is unveiled, we will likely see the bloodline of person's come forth that have the birthright, or you could say "God given ability" to assist in the Energy shift the earth and all that is in it needs. The answer is held on the interior of the cells possibly in the form of a filament that is responsible for capturing the Star Dust electrical charge.

Cycling back to the Ancient story of Adam, I must interject that "back then" there were no weeds, no insect infestations, and any number of other issues that would cause a need for any type of strenuous physical labor within the garden. This indicates that mankind came to earth in order to assist in the balance of the electrical and magnetic charge that is present in and around the earth. When Adam listened to the voice(s) of the industries of mankind, the original assignment for Adam was altered and out of the garden he went! The Star Dust within the cells became damaged and Souls began to die.

The influence of static electricity on the human cells must be resolved in order for the Adam Status to return and for the earth, along with mankind, to flourish.

Genesis 2:15-18: The Lord God took the man and placed him in the Garden of Eden to work it and watch over it. And the Lord God commanded the man, "You are free to eat from any tree of the garden, but you must not eat from the tree of the knowledge of good and evil, for on the day you eat from it, you will certainly die." (HCS)

1 Corinthians 15:44-47: ...If there is a natural body, there is also a spiritual body. So it is written: The first man Adam became a living being, the last Adam became a life-giving Spirit. However, the spiritual is not first but the natural, then the spiritual. The first man was from the earth and made of dust; the second man is from heaven. (HCS)

Chapter VI

RESURRECTION THROUGH THE BLOOD

Blood is the one element human effort has been unable to duplicate. There is too much to be learned about the wholeness of blood for anyone to successfully duplicate it, particularly where a component of Soul is involved. The life of the Soul originates from the Heavens/cosmos and cannot be matched. Blood has the capability to record everything it is exposed to. Every action taken, outfit worn, noise heard, eyes cast upon and so on is recorded and filed within the blood chemistry. Sections of the recorded information pass on to the descendant.

Sound Bites

Blood carries thousands upon thousands of tiny sound bites that surf through veins. These tiny sound bites play out from the instant they are initiated in the fetus and throughout the individual's life. The sound bites I'm referring to often show up in blood testing typically done through a physician's office or clinic. Those test results that reveal blood sugar irregularity, liver stress, kidney malfunction and so forth, are the sound bites of the lives lived by our ancestors or, in some instances, the toxic environment we ourselves have been exposed to. Sound bites can play out as an emotion, personality, or an actual disease, disability or discomfort.

I've referred to these sound bites in the past as frequencies or vibrations that become recorded in the blood; an activated sound bite might look like this:

> Grandpa experienced trauma while serving on the battlefield during his time in the military. That trauma recorded in Grandpa's blood cells. Grandpa was a young man when this took place and after the military service he returned to his home country and married. He and his wife had children and eventually grandchildren. One grandchild was born with hearing impairment and tinnitus, and experienced periodic emotional upsets. How did this grandchild, who is still quite young and had little experience in the world end up with these physical issues? The sound bites from Grandpa's experience in the military, i.e., trauma and the sound of helicopter blades chopping through the airspace, trickled down the generational line and was made manifest in a grandchild. Not all grandchildren experience the military sound bites; it's all a roll of the dice with respect to which sound bites are received at the time of conception.

Those sound bites can be erased, similar to how one would delete messages from their cell phone. A scientific explanation for this process does not exist at this time that I am aware of. Therefore, an attempt to logically process this idea may not be successful.

Microbial

What I have come to realize is genetic sound bites have a root in not only vibrations but also in bacterial infections, likely various types. Bacteria has not been removed from the blood for several generations simply because the proper cleansing process for bacteria, which comes through a specific protocol for diet and lifestyle, has not been followed and researchers have yet to discover all of the bacteria strains that currently afflict the blood. For as many antibiotics that have been prescribed and consumed it is easy to assume all bacteria would be removed from the body/blood.

If an ancestor encountered a bacteria from contaminated water and a remedy (herbal, prescription drug, etc.) was given to aid in the recovery of the individual yet the bacteria simply changed its structure of identity rather than died off and became engrained in the blood. The bacteria is no longer in a form that irritated the stomach region but is now hidden in the depths of the blood chemistry, as though the remedy applied to kill off the bacteria simply pushed the bacteria into a new location after taking on a new and different form. That trace of bacteria passes through the blood to the next generation yet manifesting as issues of the stomach, stomach pains, digestion upsets, stomach cancer, and so forth, under the radar of discovery as a bacteria. Prescription drugs have had little influence on keeping bacteria in the body at bay. It appears the prescription drugs relied on to remove a bacterial infection have only caused a change in the identity of the bacteria on some level and pushed the bacteria into the blood, now being called genetic mutation.

I share what I have come to know while having experienced many sound bites from three and four generations back that included cigarette smoking, alcoholism, sexual abuse of a child, military exposure, to name a few, none of which I was personally involved in. Meditation did not resolve the hand-me-down sound bites; therapies of various forms (acupuncture, herbal supplements, and so on) did not resolve the sound bites they merely helped me get through some of the symptoms. So what is it that erases the harmful sound bites and allows healthy cells and blood plasma to play a healthy tune?

Daily Bread

Mark 14: 22-25: As they were eating, He took bread, blessed and broke it, gave it to them and said, "Take it; this is My body." Then He took a cup, and after giving thanks, He gave it to them, and so they all drank from it. He said to them, "This is My blood that establishes the covenant; it is shed for many. I assure you: I will no longer drink of the fruit of the vine until that day when I drink it in a new way in the kingdom of God." (HCS)

First we need to interpret what is being said in the verse above. 1) Jesus is a representation of salvation (rescue). Rescue from what? Disease that has originated in the blood. The sound bites I describe are referred to as sin in Scripture. In order to erase the sin and be protected by the Covenant (promise of freedom from distress) we must partake of bread that is without leavening (Exodus 29:2; 34:18; Mark 14:12). The bread is to be broken, not cut with a knife. To use a knife (sword) implies the act of being cut off or removed from. 2) "My" body is a reference to an act that takes place in the physical body having to do with removal of or freedom from an ailment. 3) Reference to blood indicates there is an influence to the blood when the bread is properly prepared and eaten. 4) Fruit from the vine is pure Concord grape juice.

To interpret or assume the reference to wine is literal is incorrect. Wine creates a heat inside the body. Remember the heat + water = condensation analogy? God would never give an instruction to consume something that was altered by human efforts that could be potentially harmful. Alcohol has a harmful influence on the cells, aside from the fact there is a potential for addiction. A reference to wine in Scripture is a reference to blood or, a process of change that comes about over time. Scripture repeatedly expresses the importance of fresh foods. Any food carried over to the next day was to be thrown out, with the day before Sabbath being the only exception to this rule. This rule would apply to the drink as well. Wine is a result of fermentation, an aging process, a cousin to yeast.

The story of Jesus changing the water to wine is indicative of a change on the inside of the body through a process of time. This change comes through the blood.

When we add drinking the grape juice to eating the daily bread, we get what is known as Communion. Prefix "Com:" with or together. "Union:" join; unity. Joining the juice with the bread invites a power from Heaven, the cosmos, to unit with us.

There is a chemical response in the blood when wheat bread and Concord grape juice are consumed together, and yet alone - no other foods to be consumed at the time of this Communion. The physical body becomes glorified, meaning without harmful levels of sound bites/sin, when bread and Concord grape juice are consumed together on a daily basis. Sin takes up residence in the blood, not in the mind; sin may influence the mind but it does not reside there. Unleavened bread and Concord grape juice is a remedy for "sin."

An additional reference:

Our Father, whom art in Heaven, hallowed be Thy name
Thy Kingdom come Thy will be done on earth as it is in
* Heaven*
Give us this day our daily bread and forgive us our
trespasses as we forgive those who have trespassed
* against us*
Lead us not into temptation but deliver us from evil
For Thine is the Kingdom and the Power and the Glory
* forever.*
Amen.

What's is the prayer really saying?

<u>Our Father, whom art in Heaven, hallowed be Thy name</u>: The Father represents a Superior Power. Some may call this Superior Power God or Universe. Using the example of an earthly Father, Father represents someone who teaches, provides, protects (or should). *Superior Power that has an element of protection.

<u>Whom art in Heaven</u>: Addresses the fact that this Superior Power who teaches us, leads us, provides for us, not stating what is provided nor to what measure; and gives a level of protection, exists in the atmosphere, clouds or, what is most commonly called, Heaven. *A Superior Power that is in the upper atmosphere called Heaven.

<u>Hallowed be Thy Name</u>: References the greatness; the magnitude of the entity described in the previous phrase. Hallowed means great, revered, honored. *Respected; revered.

<u>Thy Kingdom come Thy will be done on earth as it is in Heaven</u>: The Superior Power that has ownership over a realm called a Kingdom is petitioned to grant or perform in a likeness that reflects what exists in the Heaven Kingdom. That Heaven Kingdom is up there, out there, in the upper atmosphere and the prayer calls for it to be reflected amongst or connect with those on earth.

One might ask what needs to take place "down here" on earth in order to be granted the presence of or interaction with this Superior Power. An act must be taken in order to create an atmosphere acceptable or to extend an acceptable invitation for the presence of that Superior Power to visit earth.

<u>Give us this day, our daily bread</u>: This is referencing literal bread, not money. There is a chemical element held within wheat bread that triggers an invitation for the Superior Power to pay us a visit. See, Genesis 41:6-7, 22-23; Deuteronomy 23:25, and other Scriptures that reference "heads of grain." *Daily we are to consume a portion of unleavened bread, which provides the signal necessary to invite the Superior Power from the Heavens.

What will this daily bread achieve in addition to signaling the Superior Power to visit us?

<u>and forgive us our trespasses as we forgive those who have trespassed against us</u>: a trespass is a violation or sin; a sin is a harmful vibration that has attached to us, to our body (in the blood). Those who have trespassed against us would be ancestors who failed to practice the proper protocol(s) required to cleanse the sin (genetic sound bites) out of their bodies. Those sins pass through the bloodline depositing the "sins of the fathers (ancestors) unto the third and fourth generations." In order to clean

out the sin(s), one must partake of a portion of unleavened bread on a daily basis. *A cancelling influence activated through a chemical reaction within the body by the bread, coupled with contact with the Superior Power.

Lead us not into temptation but deliver us from evil: The bread is a cleansing element and also a form of prevention that aids in erasing the genetic sound bites and toxic environments encountered throughout a day that can afflict blood cells.

For Thine is the Kingdom and the power and the glory forever: There is a level of power that comes from the Heaven Kingdom to our blood when we consume bread. The Glory, or being Glorified, comes through the consumption of unleavened bread when joined with the practices necessary to activate it.

There are some additional regulations sprinkled throughout Scripture and some not in Scripture that must be applied to the Daily Bread.

1) No fruit is to be eaten with bread. Eat fruits and grains at least 1-2 hours apart. The only fruit and form in which it should be consumed when eating bread is pure, organic Concord Grape Juice or Concord Grape Preserves.
2) Bread (or tortilla) should be made fresh daily, unleavened. (Do the best you can.) No crackers! Olive oil is to be used; no canola oil, vegetable oil, shortening, or other similar replacement.

Once I implemented eating unleavened bread and drinking organic Concord grape juice, the infection markers in my blood declined rapidly.

Elevating the blood glucose was another interesting factor in my journey. My diet evolved into unleavened tortillas made with organic flour, olive oil, Celtic salt and water, eaten with Concord grape juice in the evening; fresh fruits or a few select vegetables at noon and breakfast would consist of organic Cream of Wheat with pure maple syrup, more carbohydrate. Carbohydrates and fruit sugars became my diet. Exactly what many healthcare professionals will tell you to stay away from.

The implementation of Celtic salt resulted in my ability to eliminate the iodine supplement I had taken for thyroid support. Elimination of harmful food combinations and yeast, that can result in the production of harmful chemical gas and bacteria within the body proved to be valuable.

Chapter VII

MAKING IT CLEAN

Matthew 7:14: How narrow is the gate and difficult the road that leads to life, and few find it. (HCS)

It is my prayer that the protocols shared will benefit others and bring change to current situations one may be experiencing and bring forth healthy generations in the future. When life is put back into the order God designed, the health of the physical body will manifest as prosperous and full of vitality.

I'm known for my attention to detail and that certainly did not lack in this journey. Once I became aware of a need for change in a particular area, I changed according to the information and perception I had and made any necessary adjustments as I went along. I never stepped out of a protocol, going back to how things were done prior. In order to make progress and escape the ever approaching "boogie man" I knew my steps must be ordered in one direction, not giving way to two steps forward, one step back. Not all changes, eliminations or additions were easy and a handful of them went counter-clockwise to traditions or customs. Relationships were stressed or dissolved simply because others did not understand why I was doing/not doing certain things and coming up with a logical answer to their questions was challenging. Many times I did not know at the initiation of a change why I was doing it or what the result would be. Still I remained steadfast in my determination to reach a life of freedom from the ever-haunting diagnosis of a cancer or other disease.

As presented, cancer can originate from the activities, lifestyles and diet of ancestors, sepsis, an excess of inflammation and a whole host of other things. Once a genetic sound bite is present for a cancer and the individual encounters a situation that knocks on the door of the mutation, the cancer is activated.

Different types of cancer will respond with various symptoms being experienced and last for various durations of time. Recovery and change from a genetic initiated cancer, or any other cancer, is a slow, progressive process. The genetic sound bites must be erased in order to eliminate a possible reoccurrence. Dependant upon the current condition of the patient, the level of discipline applied and changes implemented, recovery and elimination of cancer can take anywhere from three to six years. At the time of this writing, my journey is soon approaching its fourth year.

The goal is to reduce exposure to EMF/EMR, static electricity, stressful environments, excess heat or cold, and toxins. I eliminated all television and had very little exposure to a cell phone or computer, which is not always possible. Rinsing in the shower each morning and evening will help reduce the influence of static electricity on the cells. The more protection you can provide for the cells the quicker new healthy cells can take action and recover the health of the body.

Incorporating the following lifestyle, fashion, dietary and environmental protocols and adjustments will aid the body in eliminating cancer and underlying infections, and lessen the chances of a repeated incident of cancer(s). When appropriate, professional medical intervention should be considered in addition to the protocols listed herein.

The physical body must have the proper amount of electrical activity in order to function optimally and to aid in the elimination of the cycle of cancer cells and any underlying infection. Interruptions in or over-burdening the electrical processes required for healthy cell regeneration and communication will hinder or prevent elimination of cancer and infections. The object is to lessen contact with items that hinder the cleansing process by impacting cells. The cells are very sensitive and while some of the protocol suggestions may seem extreme it is an effort to avoid stagnation of the progress. Each individual person will need a varying level of cleansing and what is shared is and was my personal protocol. Listen to your body.

In response to the detoxification process that will take place in the body, there will be times when a person does not feel well, feels tired or weak and symptoms in response to the cleansing process can have numerous shapes and styles. The initial 9-12 months should be had with the strictest adherence. After 12 months, some additional foods can be added which are indicated below. What should not happen is proceeding through the cleansing protocols for 12 months and returning to the prior diet and environment. The protocol is to not only eliminate distress on the body present in contaminants in the blood but to be a form of maintenance to keep any contaminates from building up throughout the remainder of days. It is no secret that the world has become overloaded with toxins that influence our body every day. These changes and additions to daily regimens take tenacity in order to stick with it.

My total calorie intake was reduced to 1,200-1,400 calories per day. Breakfast and dinner were the highest in calorie intake being of 400 calories each. Lunch was a total of 200 calories, when I ate lunch. Periodic snacking on fruits and vegetables occupied much of my food consumption. This sounds extreme and felt that way at times but it reduces the load on the blood and organs in order to allow the physical energy to focus on cleaning rather than processing. Yes, I lost weight but slowly gained weight again after the initial cleansing protocol was complete.

Maintaining an alkaline pH, an environment opposing to cancer, was and still is a benefit. Do the best you can and know that within a few months the body will begin to regain its health. It takes time!

Objective is to cleanse the blood of contaminates and allow the body to balance the chemistry within. To avoid repeating information that is easily found through a simple Google search, I have not included explanations for why particular items were incorporated or avoided. I reference Scriptures that apply when available.

THE PROTOCOLS SHARED ARE NOT OPTIONAL THEY ARE A MUST IF ELIMINATION OF INFECTION AND/OR DISEASE IS TO OCCUR. THE INFORMATION SHARED IS NOT A MEDICAL DIAGNOSIS, PRESCRIPTION OR A GUARANTEE THAT ANY SPECIFIC DISEASE OR INFECTION WILL BE ELIMINATED. STRICT ADHERANCE TO THE PROTOCOLS IS REQUIRED

AND MUST REMAIN IN PLACE THROUGHOUT THE REMAINDER OF THE INDIVIDUAL'S DAYS. SYMPTOMS MAY BE EXPERIENCED SUCH AS HEADACHE, STOMACH DISCOMFORT OR UPSET, INSOMNIA, FLUXUATIONS IN INTERNAL TEMPERATURE CAUSING CHILLS OR SWEATING, SKIN RASH, RANDOM SHORT AFFLICTIONS OF PAIN IN VARIOUS PARTS OF THE BODY, LIGHTHEADEDNESS, FATIGUE OR FEELING SLEEPY.

Chapter VIII

WHAT TO INCORPORATE

Food/Beverages:
Honey, and pure maple syrup, which also comes granulated. Do not eat honey with any yeast product; yeast and honey are not to be consumed during the Waning moon phase.

Unleavened bread made fresh daily (i.e., tortillas) for breakfast and evening meal. No bread at lunch (11:00 a.m. to 1:00 p.m.) After nine months baking powder may be incorporated into the diet.

Fresh fruit particularly berries and peaches. Fruit should not be eaten with any product made of flour, i.e., bread, pasta or pastry. (Fruit includes tomatoes, olives and avocadoes). Drink grape juice or use grape preserves ONLY when eating breads and pastas; pure maple syrup is permitted with breads.

St. DalFour fruit preserves. (Fruit preserve with no added sweeteners)

Seeds (sunflower, pumpkin, limited sesame seeds)

Sunflower seed butter.

Olive oil and sunflower seed oil.

Organic Concord Grape Juice (not concentrate). Replace water intake with Grape Juice as much as the blood glucose will allow.

Use a French press to brew roasted chicory root as a replacement for coffee and teas. Chicory is alkaline.

Fresh herbs, whole spices, not ground.

Cream of Wheat; or, steel cut oats may be eaten periodically but not daily.

After 9-12 months: add in heavy cream (cream from the herd/cow) to be used in cooking. Milk is to be from the flock (sheep or goat); cow butter may be used in limited quantifies. Cheese must be of sheep or goat. Cheese should be eaten during Waxing moon phase only. Cream may be used in the biscuits and pancakes throughout the month.

Dining/Meals:

Breakfast is to be eaten no later than 10:00 a.m.
Lunch is to be eaten between 11:00 a.m. and 1:00 p.m.;
Calorie intake at lunch is to be considerably less than
 breakfast or dinner.
Dinner can be eaten between 6:00 p.m. and twilight,
 dependant upon circumstances.

Vegetables and fruits may be eaten for lunch. No vegetables of the evening. Vegetables can cause a disruption in sleep.

If/when meats are added back into the diet after the cleansing process is complete they are to be eaten at twilight only. Meats have specific preparation and consumption guidelines that will need to be followed.

Do not eat a meal with those outside of your own household during the recovery phase. Ancient rules apply here; eating is a sacred act.

Have a set of dishes and glassware for personal use. Sharing dishes and glassware with others has an energetic influence that can result in viruses.

Clothing:

Golden Rule: Follow the Rainbow. Colors carry vibrations and those vibrations can heal or destroy whether you are wearing the color, looking at the color, living within the color. Color has been taken for granted and the clothing industry has run off course with the color pallet.

Colors can and will influence the blood; colors can hold heat inside the body or cause the body to be too cool. The clothing you wear during the day and the articles of clothing you wear at night while sleeping can have a profound influence on the way the body regulates internal temperature, sleep cycles, and refreshes itself. Colors speak to the environment we surround ourselves in; they can make things easier, more relaxed or they can make things seem more challenging. Colors, over time, will also influence the shape of the body. I am sure there is much more to what the colors can do than what I, or anyone else has discovered to date.

Beneficial colors are pastel shades. Neon colors are overpowering for the internal operations of the body and blood. If a person has internal heat in the form of an infection or genetic imprint of disease, holding heat within the body can only ignite a health issue. Black and deep, dark colors will hold the heat within the body. This heat element is not always evident on the exterior of the body. Some can experience night sweats; some have a tendency to feel cold when the temperature of the room is actually set at what should be a comfortable temperature.

Wear natural fabrics: Organic cotton, linen, alpaca, natural silk, wool. ("finely" woven; no wool with linen combinations; no bamboo). See, lifegivinglinen.com. Synthetic materials conduct static electricity.

Solid colors or small floral prints.

Women, wear dresses or skirts with a hemline to the knee or mid-shin. The circumference of a skirt carries a Symbolic value of protection; keeping people's "stuff" out of your space.

Shirts and dresses should have three-quarter to full sleeves.

Wear a belt at the waist when appropriate.

Black leather shoes with white socks are most beneficial. No nylons. 100% silk stockings are permitted when necessary. Red shoes should be worn with red clothing. Red clothing influences the blood and caution should be used with respect to what is worn in combination with red.

No black, navy, gray or white clothing. No red with black, white or green.

Undergarments should be made of organic cotton, cotton or linen and should be white or natural white during the cleansing process. No patterned fabrics.

Jeremiah 13:1: This is what the Lord said to me: "Go and buy yourself a linen undergarment and put it on, but do not put it in water." (HCS) (emphasis added)

Laundry clothing after each use including pajamas and nightgowns. Wearing articles of clothing multiple times creates opportunity for any energetic influences previously encountered to reoccur. No dry cleaning.

Hygiene:

Allowing running water to move over the body aids in removal of harmful static electricity encountered through daily activities or through the clothing worn.

Take a warm shower in the morning and in the evening.

Rinse the mouth with warm water before and after eating. This practice keeps you from "eating your words." Life and death is in the tongue and if you talk between meals, you need to rinse your mouth.

Before evening meal: Rinse the mouth and hands with warm water; wash the face with a cotton washcloth. No splashing water onto the face.

Limit lathering agents. Lathering agents irritate the thyroid. Use soaps or shampoos with little or no fragrance. Goat milk soaps are suggested.

Use a bidet and cotton bidet towels. Toilet paper leaves an energetic residue on the body. Proper cleansing and drying prevents unwanted kidney, bladder or bowel issues.

Use natural oils on the skin, i.e., almond or apricot oil. The skin conducts electricity at an increased rate when it is moist.

<u>Sleep</u>:

Why we need rest.

The Sabbath Rest

<u>Sab</u>: Person engaged in direct action to prevent a targeted activity.
<u>Bath</u>: To immerse or wash one's body.

Sabbath consists of a three day Energy reset within the body. The days mirror the death and resurrection of Christ as follows:

Friday early evening (6:00 p.m.) through Saturday 6:00 p.m.: evening is to be spent at home, including the evening meal. No gathering with others, no meals eaten out, no social activities. Seclusion is most beneficial but not always possible, particularly if you care for small children or an elderly family member.

Saturday is a continuation of Friday evening, which requires as little activity as possible. Remain in your own home and only with household members. This time is to be dedicated to being still in order for the Spirit Energy to recharge and reset the physical body (cells). A physics action takes place, joining of Spirit and Flesh (union). Too much activity interferes with this connection of Spirit and Flesh. No physical labor, work, chores, cooking (to avoid heat) or lighting candles. This is a good day for reading, puzzles or drawing. No sexual activity on Saturdays.

Scripture states that the Temple gates were opened on New Moon and Sabbath days. Gates (or gating) is a medical term referencing the activity of the cells in the body. In order for the body to receive the proper electrical charge from the cosmos, the body must be in a state of rest. The gates will then open in preparation for receiving the cosmic Energy.

Sunday is the day for relaxation, taking a nap. Light activity is permissible; cooking is permitted. The body must have rest in order to have the strength to reset and/or clean out the cells. This activity of cleansing and reset keeps the blood cells clean and the heart healthy. (Create in me a clean heart; renew a proper Spirit (Energy) within me Lord.) Again, no gathering with those outside of the immediate family unit; keep the activity to a minimum.

Monday morning introduces the changes achieved through honoring the Sabbath. Normal activity may be resumed after 6:00 a.m.

Tuesday – Friday late afternoon are days all normal activity is permitted without interference to the process of cleansing. Tuesday is the day the water is distributed to the cells/plasma creating the proper level of hydration.

Acts 17:2-3: As usual, Paul went to the synagogue and on three Sabbath days reasoned with them for the Scriptures, explaining and showing that the Messiah had to suffer and rise from the dead; "This Jesus I am proclaiming to you is the Messiah." (HCS) (emphasis added)

This Scripture mirrors the myth of the Phoenix; an act of being lowered or going down and once to the point of all things being removed (ashes), the act of rising back up occurs.

Up, showered and dressed no later than noon.

Nap (or kip) before 3:00 p.m.

To bed by 10:00 p.m. Remain inside the home after dark, no outdoor activities.

Maintain private bedchamber; limit sexual activity.

Long hair is to be in a ponytail during sleep, preventing the hair from being near the face.

<u>Upon rise from sleep</u>: rinse the mouth with water and wash the face with a cloth before consumption of food or drink.

<u>Linens</u>:

Linen bedding is the most beneficial; organic cotton and duck down are also beneficial; use pastel colors. No white bedding.

Towels and washcloths should be in pastel colors. No drying or washing the skin with white towels or white washcloths.

Fresh towels and washcloths are to be used for each shower; bedding to be laundered no less than weekly.

Cotton towels and washcloths are to be used on the skin. No scrunchies, stones or brushes.

Other:

If possible, reside outside of busy cities, away from busy highways or excessive noise and electrical power lines. Urban or country areas are best.

Maintain a clean and well-kept living environment. No clutter, dust should be kept to a minimum. Kitchen counters should be clear of clutter, dishes washed and put away prior to sleeping.

Limit pets in the home when possible.

No dirty laundry on the floor. All dirty laundry should be placed in a basket or hamper.

Practice deep breathing in through the nose, out through the mouth.

Ionic Detox Footbath. I used my Ionic Detox Footbath on a regular basis and had used it for several years. The Footbath helps reduce the stress on the lymph system as the lymph processes the toxins that are attempting to escape the body.

Mineral Stones: Tanzanite aids in counteracting cancer.

Tuning forks. Use a tuning fork, not music or recorded frequency sounds. A tuning fork will help the body process and eliminate the residue of noise encountered throughout the day. Two or three strikes of the fork at bedtime, and allow it to come to a rest should be sufficient.

Use EMF/EMR protectors.

Use air purifiers.
Reverse osmosis water for drinking.

Filtered water for bathing to reduce fluoride exposure.

Maintain an environment of 68-72 degrees Fahrenheit.

<u>It is advised that a person seek professional guidance before adding or removing any vitamin, mineral or supplement to/from their diet.</u>

Chapter IX

WHAT TO AVOID

Reading through and applying the items to AVOID into a daily regimen will feel as though all things of the world are against you. Stand firm! The goal is to eliminate as much exposure to static electricity and toxins as possible in order for the blood/cells to heal.

John 15:18-19: If the world hates you, understand that it hated Me before it hated you. If you were of the world, the world would love you as its own. However, because you are not of the world, but I have chosen you out of it, the world hates you. (HCS)

Food/Beverages:
Consuming numerous foods at one time can cause excess heat, use of excess energy to digest the food and though not yet proven can result in potential unwanted chemical reactions. To clean the blood, try to keep the diet simple with single foods or limited food combinations.

No alcohol or alcoholic beverages.

No vinegars or condiments. Celtic salt or Redmond's salt is permitted.

No artificial food coloring or flavors.

No dried herbs. Fresh herbs carry more benefit than dried.

No hot peppers, salsas or sauces during the cleansing period. These items add heat to the interior of the body.

No yeast and other leavening agents such as baking soda and baking powder for at least nine months. After nine months, baking powder may be incorporated into the diet.

No breads that are cut with a knife. Scriptures describe the act of cutting with a knife as being Symbolic of being separated from the Covenant.

No cane sugars, beet sugars, corn syrups or sweeteners. Sugars from plants that require large amounts of water will activate thirst for water or accumulation of fluid within the body.

No Xylitol and other artificial sweeteners. Check toothpaste ingredients.

No beans, lentils, including peanuts, meat, poultry, fish, seafood.

Genesis 9:3-5: Everything that lives and moves will be food for you. Just as I gave you the green plants, I now give you everything. But you must not eat meat that has its lifeblood still in it. And for your lifeblood I will surely demand an accounting. I will demand an accounting from every animal. And from each man, too, I will demand an accounting for the life of his fellow man. (NIV)

Consumption of meat is permissible after the cleansing process, with a caveat that one should understand consuming meat will influence the blood and getting out of this life without disease is unlikely.

No peanut butter or peanuts. Peanuts are in the mold family.

No chocolate.

No vegetable oil, peanut oil, coconut oil, shortening, corn oil or imitation butters.

No citrus.

No dairy, including eggs.

No coffee or teas. Coffee and tea have caffeine and mold.

Avoid drinking excessive amounts of water. Water can interrupt the electrical activity of the cells and can produce a form of condensation when added to excessive heat within the body due to infection or cancers. Slowly reduce water consumption, replacing hydration with pure fruit juices and fresh fruits when possible. According to John 4:13, drinking water results in being thirsty. No carbonated drinks, including waters.

John 4:13-14: Jesus said, "Everyone who drinks from this water will get thirsty again. But, whomever drinks from the water that I will give him will never get thirsty again, ever! In fact, the water I will give him will become a well of water springing up within him for eternal life." (HCS)

No food or beverage prepared in a microwave.

Dining/Meals:

No restaurant foods. People handling or making your food highlights a risk of cellular information transfers.

No buffet or potluck style meals. Combining numerous food types is a detriment.

Clothing:

No synthetic materials. (Rayon, Polyester, Acrylic, Nylon), denim, flannels or fleece. Synthetic materials result in static electricity that interferes with the cells.

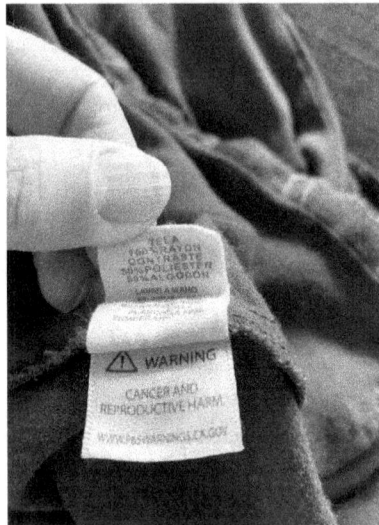

Tag sewn in collar of a casual button down shirt:
"WARNING! CANCER AND REPRODUCTIVE HARM"

Many clothing restrictions are in place to protect the meridian junctures and points in the body. This helps protect the body from receiving unwanted electrical activity that can be in the environment, including what may come through to you from another person.

No fabrics with stripes, polka dots, neon, fringe, plaid, pleats, tie-dye or large flower prints; no writing on clothing or hats.

No holes or tears in clothing.

No uneven or unfinished hemlines.

No hats made of synthetic materials or paper.

No shorts or mini-skirts.

No sleeveless shirts or dresses.

No tennis shoes or sandals; no exposed toes.

No lace across the chest. Lace across the chest influences the lymph drainage.

No costume jewelry. Plastics, glass and metals attract harmful influences. Wear authentic gemstones, gold or silver.

Hygiene:

No bathtubs or sitting in water.

No fluoride.

No antiperspirant; hair spray; lotion; cream or rubbing alcohol.

No electric toothbrushes or vigorous brushing of the teeth. Use a soft bristle toothbrush such as a natural bamboo. Avoid over stimulating the teeth.

No cosmetics. These items not only have chemicals, but eventually alter the facial features.

Sleep:

No open windows during nighttime hours in order to prevent large fluctuations in temperature.

Room should be dark; blinds closed.

Linens and Bedding:

Eliminate all synthetic bedding, pillows, and mattresses. No blankets with satin edge binding. These items create static electricity interference.

No metal or iron bed frames. Possibility of conduction of electricity if positioned near electrical outlets or electrical appliances.

Static Electricity:

Avoid all electronics, including television, all hand-held electronic devices; cell phone towers; power stations or power lines.

No electrical devices near the bed or other area for sleep.

Avoid gasoline and gasoline stations.

Very limited, preferably no travel. (Vehicle, train, bus, airplanes, motorcycles, ATVs)

No blooming plants or fresh flowers. Limit houseplants.

Live plants and the colors they display can interfere with the cell healing process.

Noise Pollution:

Vibration has an impact on the brain, particularly noise that comes through speakers or headphones.

No excessive noise. (concerts; speakers that project all forms of sound)

No music, in all forms, particularly that which comes through speakers. (May be incorporated after recovery).

No public gatherings, including school, religious meetings, social events, sporting events, holiday parties, and so forth; avoid crowds. Large crowds produce static electricity and excess noise. Numerous Symbolic influences involved here.

Toxins:

No chemicals; herbicides; pesticides; colognes; perfumes; fragrance; harsh detergents or cleaners (including vinegar); paints.

Avoid cigarette, cigar, and vaping smoke.

Eliminate all use of plastics: plastic bags or containers, drinking straws, plastic utensils, to-go cups; Teflon, aluminum cans and foil.

No nail polishes or nail salons.

<u>Other</u>:

No physical manipulation through chiropractic, acupuncture, massage or other therapies that involve manipulation of the electrical activity in the body.

No exercise or sports activity outside of general daily activities.

No camping or sleeping outdoors.

Avoid being in the rain or walking through wet pavement or puddles.

No excessive heat or cold exposure.

No hair salons, hair dyes or other chemical treatment to the hair. No hair dryers or blow dryers to the head.

No direct sunlight, without a hat covering the head. Try to avoid sunlight exposure for extended periods of time.

No cold showers; swimming pools or hot tubs.

No paper towels, paper napkins, paper plates, toilet paper or facial tissue.

<u>II Peter 2:2</u>: Many will follow their unrestrained ways, and the way of truth will be blasphemed because of them. (HCS)

Chapter X

RECIPES

Chemical Free Mouthwash: Mix 1 Quart distilled water, sea salt and a few drops of Cinnamon Bark essential oil. Use desired amount to rinse the mouth after brushing.

Tortillas: 2 Cups Bread or All Purpose Flour, 3 Tablespoon Olive Oil, 1 Teaspoon Celtic Salt, ¾-1 Cup hot water. Drizzle oil into flour and salt mixture while using a hand to incorporate the oil into the flour. Slowly add water to the flour and oil mixture mixing with the hand in a clockwise direction as the water is slowly added. Once a sticky dough is achieved, place dough onto a floured surface and knead for five minutes; tuck dough into a ball, cover with a light covering of olive oil and cover with a towel and let rest for 20 minutes. After resting, turn the dough onto the floured surface and knead 2-3 turns then pull small portions of dough and make into a ball by tucking the dough creating a golf ball sized portion. Once the dough has been formed into balls, place one ball at a time onto the floured surface and roll out with a wood rolling pin, turning the dough as you roll – roll, turn, roll, turn, continuing until the dough is paper thin, set aside. Roll each ball of dough in preparation for cooking, cover with a towel.

Cook dough on a griddle at 375 degrees Fahrenheit. When dough bubbles it is ready to be turned over; leave 2nd side of dough on griddle for 15-30 seconds, just long enough for the bubbled areas to become slightly browned. DO NOT SUBSTITUTE THE OLIVE OIL WITH ANOTHER OIL OR BUTTER.

AFTER 12 MONTHS:

Biscuits: 1 Cup Bread or All Purpose Flour, 1½ Teaspoon Baking Powder, 2 Tablespoons granulated Pure Maple Sugar, ½ Teaspoon Celtic Salt, enough Heavy Whipping Cream to make dough sticky. Mix dry ingredients and then add whipping cream to make a consistency of sticky dough. Drop dough by desired spoonful onto parchment paper lined baking sheet and bake at 425 degrees Fahrenheit for approximately 15-20 minutes. Serve with Concord Grape Preserves. You may add fresh copped herbs to the dough for flavor. DO NOT SUBSTITUTE THE GRANULATED MAPLE SUGAR WITH ANOTHER SWEETENER. BAKING POWDER SHOULD BE A SOURCE OF STARCH FROM CASSAVA OR POTATO.

Pancakes: 1 Cup Bread or All Purpose Flour, 2 Tablespoons Pure Maple sugar, 1 Teaspoon Baking Powder, ¼ Teaspoon Celtic Salt, 2 Tablespoons Heavy Whipping Cream, water to the consistency you desire. Cook on griddle at 350 degrees Fahrenheit. DO NOT SUBSTITUTE THE GRANULATED MAPLE SUGAR WITH ANY OTHER SWEETENER. BAKING POWDER SHOULD BE A SOURCE OF STARCH FROM CASSAVA OR POTATO.

Chapter XI

MOVING FORWARD

Exodus 3:7: Then the Lord said, "I have observed the misery of My people in Egypt, and have heard them crying out because of their oppressors, and I know about their sufferings." (HCS)

The way you cut your meat reflects the way you live. (Confucious)

Once a person has left the enslavement of worldly systems called Egypt, and the cleansing process has removed infections, inflammation and/or cancer, meats, with specifications, may be added into the diet. There are spiritual laws that must be adhered to when consuming meats. Otherwise, infections and disease can make their way back into the blood.

Food can never be too clean and meat can never be sliced too thin. (Confucious)

Exodus 12:11: Here is how you must eat it: you must be dressed for travel, your sandals on your feet, and your staff in your hand. You are to eat it in a hurry, it is the Lord's Passover. (HCS)

When there is occasion to consume meat you should be dressed appropriately during the meal. Shirt tucked in, belt around the waist, shoes on the feet. Your meal should not extend over a long period of time, creating a shorter duration of time from intake to completion of digestion. Many details for preparation and eating meats are sprinkled throughout Exodus Chapter 12 and Leviticus Chapter 6. Following the instructions will result in the "death angel" (sickness or disease) not having a reason to stop off at your residence/life.

Our bodies are to be functional and without debilitating affliction until the day we die. Apostle Peter was an example of this: He had received a message that it was time for him to depart the earth, to get his things in order and his means of transportation would swing by and pick him up.

2 Peter 1:12-15: Therefore, I will always remind you about these things, even though you know them and are established in the truth you have. I consider it right, as long as I am in this bodily tent, to wake you up with a reminder, knowing that I will soon lay aside my tent as our Lord Jesus Christ has also shown me. And I will also make every effort that you may be able to recall these things at any time after my departure. (HCS)

If it happened that way back then, it can happen that way now when the proper application to daily life is applied.

Chapter XII

DREAMS AND VISIONS

Acts 2:17-21: And it will be in the last days, says God, that I will pour out My Spirit on all humanity; then your sons and your daughters will prophesy, your young men will see visions, and your old men will dream dreams. I will even pour out My Spirit on My male and female slaves in those days, and they will prophesy. I will display wonders in the heaven above and signs on the earth below; blood and fire and a cloud of smoke. The sun will be turned to darkness and the moon to blood before the great and remarkable Day of the Lord comes. Then everyone who calls on the name of the Lord will be saved. (HCS)

Cleaning the blood of contaminates and graduating to a position of receiving cosmic Energy into the cells will advance or develop an ability to experience dreams and visions for some. The cells will begin to participate in an electric dance that will project in the form of dreams during sleep or visions during times of stillness or quiet meditation. I will encourage all dreams and visions to be documented on paper or in a computer. Receiving information months in advance of the birth of a situation is not uncommon and can be challenging to interpret but extremely valuable. Keeping a good record of the information received can assist in life events or decisions that may be encountered later down the road. Many times a dream or vision is a movie clip of a genetic message the cells are transcribing. Every word, every number, and every movie displayed before your eyes has a meaning. Treat them as though they were gold.

CONCLUSION

<u>STEPPING INTO ETERNAL</u>

When I look back and all I see
Are the numerous things that had happened to me.
As I grew older I'd understand
That much of my experience was part of a big plan.
What I found in that old family tree
Was disobedience for a long history.
My health told a story of the misdeeds done
All the doing of those who were from
That old family tree that became rooted within me.

Challenged on seemingly every level
I was quickly convinced there was certainly a devil.
That devil was the ancestors' lives
That passed down to me through the old archives.
The aches, the pains and fevers too,
All medics would say is I just had the flu.
This flu did not pass as many could see
So I went to God on bended knee.
Dear God, what is it I am to do?
I cannot get rid of this persistent flu.
It's not the flu my child, you see
It is years upon years of not following Me.

Your ancestors chose to follow all men
And this for them led to sin after sin.
Those sins add up when not properly addressed
And descendants are born under great physical stress.

Follow Me and you will see
That I have a plan that will recover thee.
It takes some time and much discipline too
Don't give up and you'll pull through.
For this is what I've promised to you
The DNA can change and genetics too.

Stay still, stay quiet and out of the rush
Not many will understand and create a big fuss.
Synthetics and chemicals they all must go
All natural and organic will cause you to glow.
Toss out the black, the white and the gray
It's shades of pastels that generate the ray.

The noise, the music and large gatherings
Are damaging environments and soon you will agree.
Silence is golden and where you'll find Me
This you must do so you can succeed.

Fresh bread each day with Concord Grape Juice
As directed by Me in the Scriptures produced.
No long distance travel or overnight stays
This is for sure for quite a number of days.

The cells need rest and so will you
Adopt a nap to help you get through.
Stick with My instruction and trust in Me
While My promises are sure and will protect thee.
There's a great mystery in all this you see
For I will change you to be a reflection of Me.

♛

Izauh 61™

RESOURCES

1) Holy Bible: Holman Christian Standard;
   New International Version
2) Singlecare.com
3) CreationCalendar.com

Suggested Reading:

From Antichrist to I AM
Food For The Journey To I AM
published 2022, Harvest of Healing, LLC

www.ingramcontent.com/pod-product-compliance
Lightning Source LLC
Chambersburg PA
CBHW070125030426
42335CB00016B/2266